GET A PULSE

An Emergency Room Nurse on Burnout and Breakdown

ADAM ROZENDAAL

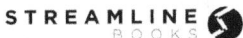

GET A PULSE

An Emergency Room Nurse on Burnout and Breakdown

Copyright © 2022 by Adam Rozendaal

All rights reserved.

No part of this book may be reproduced, distributed, or transmitted in any form or by any means, including photocopying, recording, or other electronic or mechanical methods, without the written permission from the author, except in the case of brief quotations embodied in a book review.

Cover Design by Will Severns

An Imprint of Streamline Books

www.WriteMyBooks.com

Paperback ISBN: 9-798-8378-6226-7

Hardcover ISBN:

July 11th, 2022

CONTENTS

Introduction	vii
PART 1: THE CHIEF COMPLAINT	1
Triage	9
Putting a Plan Together	15
PART 2: GATHERING INFORMATION	25
Vital Signs	29
Labs	37
Imaging	46
PART 3: CARRYING OUT THE PLAN	49
First Steps	51
Red Tape	57
PART 4: COMMUNICATION STANDARDS	67
Shades of Gray	74
Changing Shift	90
PART 5: PROBLEM BEHIND THE PAIN	97
Flavor of the Month	102
COVID-19	109
PART 6: THE MODERN-DAY HOSPITAL	125
Children & Elderly	126
Alcohol, Drugs, and Mental Health	133
Alcohol *Shudder*	133
Drugs	143
Mental Health	149
PART 7: REPEAT	159
We're Human	164
We're Fallible	165
Acknowledgments	171
About the Author	173

For any Nurse with or without a pulse.

INTRODUCTION

"Some of the most challenging moments of your life will be while you are wearing scrubs," they said. Also, some of the most rewarding and memorable ones.

In the years it took me to get my nursing degree, those that stood at the front of the classrooms made multiple comments of the difficulties of the job and yet, none of them were honest. At least not honest enough. Once or twice the instructor would throw out a 'no win' scenario about an unruly person but it was never more than discussion and it was never painted with how foul human nature can get. In their defense, they likely aren't allowed to sink to that level. If they were allowed, then each class would entail the instructors finishing a bottle of alcohol throughout the day then slapping and spitting on the class as they exited, berating them for simply being the ones who will inform future patients that the Doctor is not going to prescribe them Ativan for their anxiety after they had to be resuscitated from an overdose, no matter how severe it is.

It likely doesn't even take a shift before a fresh off the graduation stand Nurse is looking for the exit to a patient's room as the Doctor tells a husband and wife that the "bee sting" the wife checked in for when she went to pee is in fact Herpes. I wish I could tell you that it was just patients, too. That there was cohesion amongst healthcare communities. That there was an "us vs them" rally cry. It would be lovely to have the healthcare community to rally with and say, "Fuck, this sucks, doesn't it?", and have all related fields nod back and say, "Fuck yeah, bro, but you know what? We got you." That isn't the case though. Shit, I wish I could even say that Nurses have each other to turn to consistently but there is still a decent chance that a Nurse's own compatriots will be filled to the brink by a massive assortment of things that put up an impenetrable barrier to anyone else. There is a more than decent chance that their empathy has been tanked already, that they are on their 5th, 6th shift in a row and anything other than keeping the flow going is all they have to cling onto until their days off, detouring at someone else's issues would take too much energy.

One of the directions I took to for an outlet was the media. At this point, I have seen a handful of shows, listened to several podcasts, read a few books about nursing and frankly, what they are doing is serving you a huge plate of deep fried horse shit.

I realized something horribly disturbing about how nursing is portrayed on a large market scale. I realized that in the trenches, Nurses are closer to me than that of the shows, books, podcasts, etc. The shows and stories all have the same "not all heroes wear capes" bullshit theme. Like theater or a screenplay, they have the Act 1: Setup, Act 2: Struggle, and Act 3: Triumph and live to fight another day.

INTRODUCTION

Let's just start this particular journey expanding that. These forms of media go one of two ways: they contain tales of heroism with dashes of made-up drama to keep you on the edge of your seat. They are typically wrapped up with some nice message about how you should keep fighting whatever good fight there is to be fought. Some real life 'superhero' bullshit—as if 117 Marvel movies have started getting to people's heads. There may be some nods to teamwork or acknowledging a job well done by someone else, but it always circles back to the creator; it is minutes upon minutes or pages upon pages of ego inflating self-doting. Many try to reel it back in with an "I'm just like any other person" message. Or they give some juxtaposition on nursing through the lens of a person who represents health but is tormented with their own demons without a healthy handle on them.

From a mid-level standpoint, there are two basic outlines with these books, blogs, or whatever:

1. The experienced Nurse who has stood their ground against peers, protocol, or Doctors. They kept their stance with sheer grit. They write themselves into some medical drama where the sick patient who has fallen so ill that they are at the veil between life and death is brought back because said Nurse stumbled upon whatever damn piece of the puzzle was missing. They found the needle in the haystack! The patient enjoyed chamomile tea or some Witch's Brew concoction that interfered with a new medication or whatever which led to blah blah blah. Some real heroic shit.

2. *Or* the stories take place fresh out of schooling—the Nurse goes above and beyond the call of nursing to save or change a person's life. Every time they claim some story along the lines of "I found my inner strength" or "I didn't know it would be this hard", which is banter that reeks of palpable garbage.

And it certainly is garbage. Hot loads of it. Are all such books and resources like this? Of course not. But here's something for you in regards to those stories, they are all some variation of 'look how fucking cool I am'. Especially the ones that are emergency medicine based, they are pages upon pages stuffed with things like gunshot wounds, car wrecks, delivering babies, mass disasters, oh my! They might as well end with a QR code that takes you to a video of the Nurse walking away from the hospital exploding. Whenever I talk about nursing, it's more like a PSA.

If you or a loved one is considering Nursing as a career, know this: Nursing is hours on end, bending your schedule and priorities to fit the demands of (often) ungrateful patients. If there's any truth to all those nursing stories out there, it is the real struggle of being *heard* in such a hectic environment. Most Physicians are quick to counter your suggestion with something you didn't think of—something not necessarily better or worse, but something you just didn't think of in the first place. Then there is the type that simply yells at you outright, declaring that the fact you even reached out to them for anything other than a blood soaked floor after 5pm is not appropriate. Granted, that level of extreme is also typically a surgeon but a level of it exists with most Providers.

And when you *do* spend extra time on a favorable outcome for any given patient, there seems to be three or four other patients and their families you haven't seen within the hour because of successful time spent elsewhere. In fact, sometimes those families come looking for YOU! They will roam the halls like a big cat hunting its prey. It also doesn't matter the scenario in which some of them find you. In one instance, I was literally walking out of a serious trauma patient. We're talking about a vehicular accident: the person with bones sticking out, blood covering the floor, 12 people in the room whose expertise spans four medical specialties, six to eight medicines running through three to four different areas of their body, a tube in their throat in addition to a breathing machine apparatus. Only for me to turn around, and there they are . . .

That face.

A random patient's family member with a look on their baffled, traumatized face. ("Are those . . . bones?") That face that immediately speaks to the darkest parts of your soul because they are about to let you know how inattentive you've been to their loved one's need for a warm blanket.

Or in another case, my hands full of sedating medications and splinting material while a family member yells my name from 20 feet down the hall *JUST* to let me know their adult family member (my other patient), who is fully capable of holding their piss for an hour, has to go to the bathroom. All in all, nursing is running around endlessly—behind on your work, getting yelled at over trivial things, and juggling diagnoses in an effort to get people in and out of any given hospital in a sufficient manner.

And that is a small dose of reality for Nurses across America. Now allow for the *following* taste of customer service when it comes to emergency care.

Yeah, you read that right. Customer service in the ER is not just a problem, it is *way too much* of a problem in the fabric of our medical society. In all seriousness, I blame reality television. Television reinforces us with the notion that being polite and working for what you want is a distant Plan B to the dramatized way of life and career we see fleshed out on screen.

Television (as well as YouTube, social media, and the like) also reinforces the easy path of immediate gratification and that bullshit notion that "The customer is always right." How is that phrase still a thing? Everyone knows it is an absolute farce and yet, it lingers. You want your custom home built correctly, right? You want your car to have a properly installed transmission, correct? The same goes for your health and general bodily welfare.

Which brings us to the point of this book's introduction.

I spent eight years as an Emergency Nurse, and then, in (2019), moved onto the Intensive Care Unit (ICU). As of this writing, I serve as a traveling Registered Nurse (RN) for ICUs across the country. Prior to my schooling and training as a Nurse, I served as a Medic in the Army with two deployments.

All of the moves I made with my career were influenced by a logic of 'following the patient'. I would advance my knowledge of the sciences and work from the point of injury for a handful of years, then progress into the Emergency Room where a larger aspect of patient stabilization, patient care procedures and greater management with more resources exists—eventually progressing to how a patient heals through prolonged management and even more long-term organization of the critically injured. (Without getting any further into the chronology of my vocational journey). I remember being so excited to be in the Emergency Room. We're talking about the day-to-day happenings of heart attacks, strokes, out of control infections (known as sepsis), traumatic events like car accidents and gunshot injuries . . . so many other situations that present an opportunity to exercise my skills and knowledge to be light for people on their darkest day. I was jazzed!

Pump the brakes, though. Because the point of this book isn't to inspire you. It's to frighten you. You're not about to read a retelling of Florence Nightingale. You're about to read my perspective on the unnecessary complications of trying to do a good thing. The nursing Mr. Hyde behind Dr. Jekyll.

When I began working in the Emergency Room, at around the age of 27, many of my peers were in the early throws of their individual careers. My friends and I were always so curious of how one another's work lives were coming into focus. One of the most frequent questions my friends would ask me was a variation of, "Damn, man. The ER? Do you leave every shift just covered in blood?"

Not quite. Not even close. Running around covered in puke, piss, and/or shit is more accurate—which is all not so much a guarantee but a likelihood from shift to shift. Covered in sweat from the aforementioned running around for twelve hours on the other hand? *That's* the guarantee.

So with some lovely visuals in mind, let's proceed. My goal through this entire thing is to peel back and let people peek through the veil a little. At least from the perspective of nursing through critical care. I'm not going to tee you up to pass any national nursing exam but along the way if you learn a thing or two about ER or Nursing mindset along the way, splendid!

I would also like to hopefully create a little fucking empathy, empathy all around: for patients and their Nurses. Being an asshole is easy, being empathetic builds character.

The structure of accomplishing this goal is centered around the general outline of an ER & how it's run, some of the nitty gritty explained, some commonalities of an experience in the ER—highlighting both the individual on the ER side of things (in the context of this book, from a Nurse's perspective) as well as highlighting the individual on the receiving end: the *patient* side. Followed up with some straight up stories that you could hear in any given circle of ER Nurses.

Which leads us to one of modern day's giant fucking ironies: that of the impatient patient. This person is not *you*, it is all of us. We have all been the impatient patient, but this individual is partly what led me to write this book.

We'll follow the format of a common ER patient's pathway except from the Nurse's view of the internal order of operations from the beginning chief complaint through the typical obstacle course that is the human interactions of the ER and what it takes to get a patient from the entrance to their next destination. Then Repeat.

That's right. I said "repeat." If knowing the end of this book in advance—that nursing is going through hell and back each week, over and again—is enough for you to put this stack of pages down and turn the other way, by all means do so. But if you want to peel back the nursing curtain with me—behind the television screens, behind the textbooks, and behind the parental advisory stickers—then turn the page and buckle up. Because take it from me: when you forget to buckle up, things will get so fucked up you quite literally won't know which way is up.

Hi, I'm Adam.

PART 1: THE CHIEF COMPLAINT

This is where everything begins: The chief complaint.

When any patient enters the Emergency Room—unless said patient is totally unconscious—there is an "interview" that will take place at the beginning of the process. Medical professionals can't always tell, just by looking at a patient, what brought a person to them. We ask questions to determine what we call a "chief complaint." Having a chief complaint gives direction to an individual's experience in the ER. To nail down the chief complaint is to assess the key ailment we are investigating. Sometimes, in a massive traumatic event, there are several chief complaints. But barring any massive traumatic events, there are typically one or two chief complaints involved. Your body is obviously interconnected systems so yeah, a single event will affect multiple systems but what we're looking for is the event.

Generally speaking, "pain" is probably the Master Chief of chief complaints. It is attached to nearly every visit in the ER. So, I convey the following with complete sincerity: if any patient is experiencing pain, and the pain itself—no matter where on one's body—is to a point where "I can't handle the pain," then the patient is already in a tough spot when facing the staff. Nurses simply have had too much experience dealing with trauma patients to fall for the "I can't handle the pain" trope. The telling sign for a Nurse is when patients answer our follow-up question: "When did this pain begin?" Instead of days or weeks trying to endure the pain, the answer is, unfortunately, entirely too brief.

You know how when your smartphone stops working for like . . . five minutes? And you automatically wonder where the nearest smartphone repair shop is? Or, more accurately, how much a new phone in general would cost? When in reality all you need to do is turn the phone on and off again to get it working . . .

That's kind of how it is with a number of Emergency Room patients asking us to diagnose their Chief Concern.

As a matter of fact, a person with those lingering pains should first consult their primary Doctor before something becomes an "Oh, my God, I can't take this anymore" pain. Always keep your primary Doctor in the loop anyway. They can best take care of you if they are informed. But really what I'm getting at is don't wait until it is an emergency then call them - read on to learn about prevention. Over the phone at odd hours, they will refer most complaints to the ER anyway, they cannot do a true evaluation from miles away. You will also likely speak to the on-call Physician who *then* might refer someone to the Emergency Room, but overall, here's something you should know about a lot of primary Doctors: they're sick of dealing with melodramatic shit on the side. When patients call them and describe a normal ache/pain—

pain that will 99.99% of the time will dissipate after you sleep on it (remember, turning off and on the smartphone??)—the reality is we aren't in the "take two and call me in the morning" era. Many primary Doctors will send said patient to the ER "just in case."

Is there some validity in going to the ER "just in case"? Perhaps. Is there also some validity in primary Doctors sending patients to the ER in the event there *is* something wrong and instead of "sleeping on it" things get worse and someone (the primary Doctor) gets sued? Abso-fucking-lutely. In America, there are a lot of patients who . . . wait for it . . . like to sue Doctors! And because there are plenty of primary Doctors who would prefer to book their next vacation instead of getting a summons, refer their patient to the ER for nearly no matter what the patient has called the office. "Take two Aspirin and call me in the morning" is dead.

Do you see where this is all heading? On one hand, yes, the beginning of any Emergency Room process begins with an interview to diagnose the chief complaint. On the other hand, some books you might read in life kick off their first chapter with their own version of a chief complaint.

This is mine.

In about ten years of Emergency Nursing I have been face-to-face with human frailty on a nearly daily basis. The percentage of "high pain tolerance" patients actually experiencing an emergency is undoubtedly a failing test percentage. So, if a patient wants to get their interview off to a good start, they shouldn't tell an ER Nurse about how tough they are, because you're not auditioning to be a patient on a new CBS show. This also goes for people who come through the door screaming and yelling uncontrollably. At an ER, if you come in screaming and yelling that tells us you are conscious and have a functioning airway. Drama doesn't go far in this department. Typically, legitimately sick or injured people are too focused on slowing down to heal instead of trying to win a damn Oscar for "Best Supporting Ruptured Appendix".

Many Nurses become Nurses because they appreciate the human influence behind injury and illness. There is a very legitimate ordeal when a person is sick—and I mean *truly* sick—they internalize their situation to the point of inaction (Note: *"truly* sick" can also include a serious bodily injury). The sick or injured person doesn't put on a show or scream it from a mountaintop, they most certainly don't post that shit to social media. They compartmentalize, but intrinsically know something is wrong. The most sick people I ever cared for were stoic to their core. When people have a serious ailment, it is as though their body seems to tell them *how* and *where* they need to focus their energy. Their body is fighting off something and needs to mend. Babies are a helpful example. If a baby is quiet and doesn't have a "stranger danger" type reaction to the staff, that is a sick baby. Truly sick people and babies have no time for drama—their bodies are too focused on the ailment or injury at hand to bring excess drama into the scenario. (And for all the medical people reading this that are thinking "this fucker doesn't know what shock is," layman's book, here, remember?)

Still need some convincing to leave all (possible) drama out of the ER? One of the most memorable stories I can recall goes out to all the supposed "badasses" out there. The ones who might, in fact, have an ER Oscar to their name. After all, this story was so entertaining and memorable I decided to give it a couple pages in this book. Some pretty prime real estate, if you ask me.

It was a cold, unusually packed night in the ER where hospital rooms were full to the max. And I mean to the *max*. Even the "last-effort beds" were taken—beds that are known as "code beds" and reserved for people who have illness or injury and, if they don't get immediate and continuous attention, usually end in death or a vegetable state. So, when this situation arises, we either transfer patients to a sister hospital within the same network or we board them in the ER (as in room and board).

In that wild couple of hours, who was I assigned? One of the sweetest elderly ladies any Nurse could hope for as a patient, she never once lost her disposition at how busy things were. And that was a BUSY night. She was boarded for further monitoring of chest pain that didn't have any serious stand out red flags. "Boarding a patient" means you keep the patient in the ER because there are no rooms at the inn, ER Nurses do their hospital intake, perform their admission in addition to regular hospital orders—well, you do those things to the best of your ability. Boarding a patient also means confirming the parts of their medical history that were covered upon their arrival such as allergies, medical history, social history, surgical history, etc. Getting to the point, I had some time to talk with her & confirm things. When I asked her about her smoking history she told me, "Well, I used to smoke but that was only for a couple years and it was only to help me stay awake while welding airplanes together during the war."

Two things super quick 1) Smoking will murder you, murder you a slow, awful manner. That's just how it is. 2) That was still one of the most badass things I had ever heard. And likely the most badass person I have ever met. She has experienced some shit in her days that has her pain scale on a whole different level. Feel free to start a petition to put that lady in charge of the pain scale. Tell her about your problems.

That night led me to an interaction with this sweet old lady who knew something about enduring *real* pain. You could hear it in her voice—years of welding planes during the war . . . it made me think about the other patients in the hospital that night. Who knows whatever the hell they were taking up those beds for—some of them legitimate, but others probably (again) could have slept it off. And there I was with Mrs. Badass in all her kind glory, thinking about her chief complaint (whether she realized it or not) and whether or not it was something that could have been prevented without those years of smoking..

Which leads to the best thing a person can do for their health: preventative medicine. For the sake of your health, from birth to dirt, preventative medicine is taking action to avert detriments if possible and adjust accordingly to lessen any sort of future ailment or injury you might still experience. Wearing a helmet and leather gear while riding a motorcycle is a great example of preventative medicine (or, stated in the introduction, wearing your seatbelt). Yeah, that wind ripping through your shirt is cool and all but you do NOT want to be the person that left a 300 ft trail of their blood and skin down the interstate because the pavement ripped through their body. Human Crayon, I believe the term is.

An even better, less graphic example is EXERCISE. An unfortunate reality of modern medicine is how little people move their bodies. After you put this book down, pay a little extra attention to news stories about exercise. Every year, like anyone is trying to keep it a secret, there are some new studies about the benefits of exercise. If you follow the trend on what they are recommending people do, you'll find the content quite comical. The headlines used to be about how exercising for 30 minutes a day or whatever will reduce your risk for heart disease by X amount. And people bitch, moan, and cry that they don't have that much time in their weekly schedule. The next study might come out saying that just *20* minutes for three to four times a week will drastically benefit your long-term health. Next year: 15 minutes of movement is good for you! Fast forward five years and our headlines might read: "PLEASE, FOR THE LOVE OF GOD, DO SOMETHING! LITERALLY ANYTHING! YOU ARE KILLING YOURSELF!"

But this project is meant to be much more than *my* chief complaint(s). Well, it's maybe mostly a chief complaint but a chief complaint with a purpose, otherwise it's just pages of complaining. I want people to learn. I want people to understand how things work in an ER because, God forbid, they should end up in the Emergency Department one day . . . they won't spew excess drama or misplaced anger on the staff who are merely trying to manage several hundred worst days of a person's life, of a family's life. As for Nurses, I want them to learn from this book as well. Especially to aspiring Nurses. Textbooks don't get dirty when teaching, and while scrolling through memes add a flair of 'reality comedy.' They don't paint a true picture of what happens inside these walls. This book is meant to do both: serve as a mortar between learning and reality.

As a Nurse, beginning one's work in the Emergency Department starts with the delusion that we might actually be helping people. Little does a new Nurse realize one is rarely mitigating emergencies through useful practices like CPR and various methods to stop the bleeding. Instead, Nurses take on a ridiculous amount of roles. You are a Nurse (of course) but you are also a teacher, a dietitian, homeopath, a respiratory therapist, a psychiatrist (honestly, I would love to see a "bridge" program where, while studying/working to become a Nurse, you fulfill a large amount of credit hours toward a degree in Psychiatry), in addition to a pharmacist, orthopedist, physical/occupational therapist, wound management; the duties flow into roles far beyond nursing and healthcare to housekeeper, negotiator, transportation coordinator.

One of the most common things I've done in my nursing career is have a conversation with patients who fortunately walk away from a car accident unscathed that I do not know where their cell phone is and I will not allow them to use my personal cell to call somewhere. Patients will spend more time arguing with me that they "always have their phone on them" than they do listening to their instructions on where to go from the ER. The fact that their phone was likely flung a hundred and fifty feet off the interstate from when they wrecked, or that maybe the Paramedics gave more attention to pulling their body out of a mangled vehicle than searching for their iPhone is too much to grasp. This is 2022, people. Maybe one of the 'takeaways' that I should reach for by writing this is to have people dial numbers in their cellphones every so often. Especially, if it is a commonly used number. That way, patients will still have a feasible way to get back home if they are ever unfortunately brought to the ER at midnight.

The ER Nurse is a "catch all" profession. Nobody in the department has any control over what comes through the doors at any given moment. In the realm of Nursing Education, it takes additional study in the area of cardiac resuscitation, pediatric emergencies, and trauma management just to be baseline competent.

Sounds simple enough? Then we can maybe move forward with an agreed chief complaint across the board: Patients, your Nurses are trying the best they can with what they have —Nurses, your *patients* deserve *patience* no matter how many Oscars they're trying to win. Yes, it can be annoying as hell but who knows the day they've had (or maybe the *life* they've endured). Because if you think assessing the chief complaint is a drama-filled experience, wait until the Initial Interview comes into play. To examine someone's, *anyone's,* history is when things get really fucked up. And spoiler alert—Nurses aren't exempt from checking their own batshit history at the door.

TRIAGE

Let me start explaining the emergency process with something you already know: The ER is not the damn grocery store checkout. Apparently, only a few people know that it is based on medical urgency since the air at an ER waiting room is filled with a regular chorus of "I've been here for hours, other people have gone in that showed up after me."

IT IS NOT first come, first served. How people are seen by the Doctors is based upon how sick or injured they are. Now, I know the act of throwing up sucks, diarrhea is the worst, and that sore throat you've been dealing with for far too long (because you can tolerate a lot of pain) is now unbearable, but guess what? As it turns out, things like heart attacks, strokes, and major traumatic events will be treated before your sniffles and sprained ankles. Why? Because time will kill you before that sprained ankle. Even in extreme cases, you might not be seen or treated first. Broken things are an excellent reason to come to the ER—a broken arm for example. Broken arms are a "looks like a duck, sounds like a duck" scenario for Nurses. You might have fallen on it and heard it and heard a *SNAP*. Naturally, someone drives you to the ER, but wouldn't you know it?! Some other asshole just had to get stabbed or shot and arrived at the ER at the same time as you . . . nuts! They are going to be seen first, especially if that type of an injury is *checks notes* literally anywhere on their body. Their injury poses a greater threat to their life.

Of course, there are little tidbits that could change the situation as things progress. Let's say the other person hurt their arm as well, and the surrounding area to the injury is otherwise normal. Or let's also say your broken arm, upon examination, shows that your arm contains two different things on either side of the break: 1) the color of said arm you are used to is darker in nature, and 2) the skin temperature is colder than you are used to near the far side of the break. These two elements mean "Oh, shit" and you just garnered a lot more attention than the other person because it shows there is an interruption in blood flow. Plain speak: you are now in a situation where you could lose your arm.

What you just read is a microcosm of a process called 'Triaging.' Triaging is taken from the French word which means 'to sort.' In the ER, we 'sort' patients with the mentality of "Who will die first." There's no sugar-coating that one. Triaging can be an extremely difficult process and takes years of experience coupled with a great deal of underlying knowledge to perform effectively. It is one of those skills that is never done perfectly. *Effective* saves lives, striving for *perfection* will get people killed.

PART 1: THE CHIEF COMPLAINT   11

Triage is so important that learning how to triage, the Day 1 Teaching on how to do triage is broken down into some kindergarten-level ABC shit: Airway, Breathing, Circulation. Now . . . it is actually C-A-B or H-A-B-C, but in the military, it's actually called M-A-R-C-H. There are several kinds of acronyms that speak to the same idea, so if you are trained in emergency medicine and I didn't mention the one you use, deal with it or write your own book. The point is these acronyms teach to observe for signs of clues to life threatening or major bodily complications because the point of triage is to determine, within split seconds, which person(out of a sometimes quite large group) is dead if nothing is done soon, to look for threats to a person's life, limb, or eyesight.

Then, which injuries or illnesses amongst the people not suspected of immediate deterioration will deteriorate first? It gets dicey easily, too, a person will be killed by a massive amount of blood loss before a compromised airway . . . but that is a path that will get a little too into the weeds for the purpose here. Also, hence the teaching tool.

Hemorrhage, Airway, Breathing, Circulation, you see, through the millennia of providing care to sick and injured people, with all of our advancements, we simplified it down to those little letters as being the most important things to keep a keen eye on. Really, it is so that when the shit hits the fan, you have a place to center yourself—you can collect yourself and move forward accordingly. Pragmatically, as a Registered Nurse, it might sound like this, "Shit, fuck, shit, I don't know what to do . . . oh, yeah! ABCs. HEMORRHAGE. Is there blood everywhere? Check. Now *AIRWAY*. Is air moving through my patient's body? Check. *BREATHING*. How close to normal does this movement of air appear? Is their chest moving as one solid piece, and are they exerting any extra muscles while breathing? Check. *CIRCULATION.* Are they a different color than expected? That blood that should be going around and around inside the body—is it going around but then out of the body? Check."

All other owies and boo-boos can wait a minute. Yes, yes, I know . . . sometimes those wounds are super painful. Think of this: *every* pain a newborn baby feels is literally the worst pain of its life. Some people simply grow up without raising that threshold.

But let me put it to you like this.

If you put a bandage on a wound, that is called 'dressing the wound.' And it can be time consuming, as these injuries soak up our attention. They draw our eyes to them if they are profound and nagging enough. I mean, if a man walks up to you with his arm bending in a manner that it should not be bending, you are going to gawk at that shit! Am I right or am I right? ... I'm right. BUT if you give that ugly break too much attention, you might not realize if your patient is breathing effectively . . . if at all. Or you won't pay attention to their adequate heart rate (or lack thereof) and blood pressure. In summary, if you never keep a keen eye for the more serious, quieter issue . . . well, you may have dressed a patient up all nice and pretty just to send them to the morgue.

SO, for any future patient out there sitting in triage, bitching about how something-or-other hurts and you cannot take it anymore . . . guess what? Most Nurses are tuning out such sob stories and the events leading up to the ER. BUT, they *are* still doing something quite important. Mental notes are being made, notes like the fact you have an intact airway and are in fact passing air effectively through it. You would not be able to do that if you were choking or dying from blood loss.

There are a tremendous amount of asterisks to triage but do remember the takeaway, triage is to make a rapid call on who will have a bad day versus who will have no more days based upon how soon they are seen by the full complement of the ER.

Now, it's worth making a special note on *bleeding*. People can bleed a lot before it comes to the attention of a Nurse. Our bodies fight to survive and make changes to try their best to remain 'normal' through abnormal events. It might take a little while for a person in serious trouble to display serious ailment(s), *especially* if the offending bleed is on the inside. In addition, consider the following. Weather patterns do play a factor in a multitude of ways. But bleeding presents a unique challenge depending on the season. People wear a lot of clothes in the winter and Eddie Bauer (or North Face or Carhartt or your brand of choice) absorbs that shit blood pretty impressively. You could have a very serious injury but not an obvious display because your extra layers are taking in all the blood. Also, unless you are trying to 'make it' on TikTok and receive a spray tan every other week, then through the winter months you probably are pretty pale. So, sometimes that color change is less apparent.

In the ER, Nurses constantly monitor what is known as your mental status. Are you acting appropriately? Do you seem fidgety or distressed? You see, a deficiency in any of your ABCs could alter your mental state. Not as easy a job as you would think to determine. When someone says some really ridiculous shit, I need to determine if that person is acting all sack-of-hammers because they are concussed, or if they are not getting oxygen and/or blood to their brain, if there is a substance causing them to slur their words or maybe they are simply the type of person where when people describe them, they begin with "bless his heart." It is all a part of triage.

However, explaining that reality to people about how our processes work never goes well. Think I'm exaggerating? Take a look at some Google Reviews of any ER and see how many bad reviews are because of the general wait time(s) during triage—the general population's chief complaint of an ER is the wait. Any given individual is numero uno (in their eyes) and everyone else can suck it. The act of "waiting" is the most common reason Nurses get yelled at. And typically, it's common that Providers (Doctor, Nurse Practitioner, Physician Assistant) rarely get such treatment—they're the hero in this equation, and the person the patient came to see. Until the Provider enters the mix, most Nurses are mere obstacles in flesh form.

Nurses get yelled at during triage from start to finish. As mentioned previously, triaging is a skill that even battle-tested professionals take years to cultivate—so no, I don't expect a patient to totally understand the fact, even though *they're* hurting or someone they love is hurting, there are others whose needs might come before their own. All of which is an understandable recipe for an angry mob.

I know, I know . . . I've mostly painted a picture of a room full of people being ignored. But that is just not the case—triage rooms have a constant circulation of ER Techs, EMTs or additional RNs to keep any visitor as updated as possible. My hope is that this understanding of triage makes the angry ER mob, well, a little less angry.

The "frustrating wait," as a chief complaint, also isn't resolved once a patient is inside the department. Giving increased attention to a more critically ill patient is a 24hrs a day ordeal. A familiar refrain—"Well, I am in the EMERGENCY ROOM aren't I?"—gets tiresome to hear for any Nurse. In a perfect world we could tell them, "That doesn't mean you're experiencing an EMERGENCY" and match their annoyance. But such words, as we know, would only lead to more of those ugly Google Reviews. As previously mentioned, Nurses understand some patients have real pain and many patients have zero patience. In either case, a sore back is just not as important as someone who can't breathe.

In other words, many patients treat the Emergency Room like an Applebee's. Once they feel better, it's "Check, please!" with the "please" rarely making an appearance. And if it does, Nurses and staff rarely sense any true gratitude. Therefore, we're going to round out Part 1 with a little recap of an ER triage experience from start to finish. In doing so, let's cultivate a little more appreciation all around. A little less complaining and a little more training. A little less Applebee's, a little more Hospital—because the people trying to funnel humans in and out really do have the patient's best interests in mind.

PUTTING A PLAN TOGETHER

At the initial greeting and observation of a patient, Nurses have one question in mind as we stand across from whatever "ailing" bag of bones decided that day was the day to get their rash checked out by a Doctor: where on a scale of "sick or not sick" does this person sit? From that moment on, our goal is to put a plan together on how to best manage their complaint. The ER needs to be a continual motion machine. Any moment could be a person's legitimately worst day ever, so we don't like to get backlogged any more than the natural process calls for. So, when you go to the ER, you will be asked a quite simple question:

"What brings you into the ER today?"

The answer to that question already begins a mental workup by the ER team, so for the love of whatever you believe in, let's not (patient *or* Nurse) make this part harder than it needs to be. All the patient needs to do is keep the answer simple. We completely understand that you are a whole person, the intent is not to reduce you to a single thing. But there are already a hundred thousand ways to improve healthcare and streamlining the ER is certainly one of them. If you want to spend an afternoon being recognized for the individual you are, join a group.

As for the ER? Explain the problem or area of your body where you are experiencing pain or discomfort. Items such as: "I can't catch my breath" or "I fell down and now (fill in the blank) hurts" or maybe the ole *points to elbow* that should in no way be bending that direction and we'll get the basic idea of what brought you in. Unfortunately, patients don't always respond in such simple terms. People often respond like they're bullshitting their way through a question on the written portion of the SAT or ACT test. For instance . . .

"The other night, just last week, there was lightning outside and my family came over—they sometimes come to check on me, and so they came over because of the lightning and all. You see, we have these boxes on the telephone poles outside . . . oh, gosh, what are those things called? But the boxes are high up there. You know what I mean. So, my family showed up and they brought my cousin's girlfriend with them. It was pretty unusual because my cousin and his girlfriend have only been dating off-and-on. They seem like they are in a good place now, so I was happy she came to visit. Well, the reason my cousin came is because he's good at home repair and generally just nice to have around. I wondered if he might be useful because of those boxes on the telephone poles . . ."

At that point, I tried (um, I mean "would try") to interject to get them back on track—remember, that simple question of "What brought you into the ER?"—with a clarifying question such as "So you got hurt helping your cousin with home repair? What exactly brings you to the ER?"

The story just continued (I mean, might perhaps continue), "Oh, no I wasn't helping him with the repairs. HOWEVER, funny you ask because one time we *were* working in the backyard when . . . "

SO, if you answer any Nurse's question by taking a deep breath, you're off to a bad start. If you possess the time of day to give us a 10-minute story that may or may not find its way to a chief complaint, then you should have had the time to either make an appointment with your family Doctor or Urgent Care instead. There is a busy ER we're trying to keep afloat, and our goal is simply to attain enough pertinent information to relay to the Provider. The ER is not like a TV drama—there is not some obscure detail to 'break the case.' If you assume the position of detective, many Nurses might resort to the ever-powerful: "In one single sentence, tell me why you are here."

The following is an example of how business should operate in an effort to keep the ER moving.

"I fell off my bike and now my arm hurts."

Bravo! Great answer. The solid quick-answer response isn't

even limited to singular, traumatic events nor is it isolating body systems. A person can even have two complaints without telling us about what happened over Christmas. Just tell us what ailment(s) brought you into this building and we will fall back on our years of schooling and experience to understand that bodily systems are connected. Check it out:

"I've been throwing up for the last two days."

OR

"I've been getting dizzy off-and-on since this morning."

OR

"My side hurts out of nowhere, and it makes it hard to breathe."

See, it can be short and sweet for anything. Even a catastrophic event like a high speed car crash can be simplified. Trauma Doctors and Nurses take additional training to understand the consequences and interconnected dynamics of all sorts of chief complaints. So, once more, for the love of all those that came before you, we don't need to know the whole series of unfortunate events that lead to an avocado getting stuck in your asshole, we just need to know that there is indeed an avocado in your asshole. One that you presumably would like removed.

The ER is a department of contradictions. An ideal "short" triage period is paired with the unfortunate "long" story being told to any Nurse on call. People want in, they want fixed, and they want to move the fuck on. But yet, somewhere burrowed inside is a person's psyche is the need to fucking talk about their own self. People will sit in ER rooms and stew with anger over their two-hour visit, yet once their time comes for a face-to-face with staff, they're ready to chat over afternoon coffee.

But here's a little inside baseball for you: the ER has trackers that show Nurses and staff not only *how long* you have been in the department, but how long ago certain events took place such as: when you got to your room, when you entered Computed Tomography (CT), when labs were drawn, etc. So, when you complain about the amount of time you've been waiting or the crazy ER journey you've been on, know that we'd be more than happy to fact check.

I hope the previous paragraphs are enough to enlighten an ER process done well. Should you make the experience more difficult than it needs to be? Well, then you run the risk of becoming a boomerang patient.

Boomerang patients are the ones that go home, don't feel better and head on back to the Emergency Room. Boomerang patients will sometimes visit the ER multiple times in a week because they didn't leave feeling better or their situation changed for the worse—even after a short time. Obviously, there *are* situations that warrant return. Those reasons are communicated in a patient's instructions for going home in the first place. But holy shit, good God almighty—wouldn't you know that seemingly half of America will come back THE SAME DAY after being diagnosed with Strep Throat because they aren't feeling better. Or after a day or two from a major injury because it "still hurts . . . " And so we come full circle to the chief complaint: mine and theirs.

So let's move on from the chief complaint and give you a taste of putting a plan together. In Part 3, we'll dive a little deeper into this "plan of action" as it relates to complications that arise on the job.

You see, when a patient makes it successfully past triage and everyone is feeling good about next steps in the ER room—patient *and* Nurse—it's time to start putting a plan together. This is also a decent place to acknowledge that our current healthcare system, in the United States of America, is for the most part a giant fucking mess. A tragic one at that. So perhaps the following Part(s) can help us all Put a Plan Together to make the healthcare system a little less . . . shitty. Nevertheless, efficiency is key in any emergency room, so my rant holds true. Let's keep this shit simple.

From there the grunt work of the Emergency Room is acting out the plan that has been put together. The unnecessary obstacles sure as shit don't stop at triage either. They actually increase, quite greatly, too. Entering this territory needs to begin with the fact that there is no such thing as a pain free option. The road to getting better is ugly. And unless you have been there before, either yourself, or there with someone, you don't know how ugly it can get. There comes a point with nearly every ER patient that is basically their boiling point. Then they boil over. They did not expect the system to look like it does. They have this imaginative scenario where as soon as they get to the hospital they are on the path towards things being lovely. So, after the wait in triage that makes waiting in the sun at Disney World seem enjoyable, the wait in the Emergency Room itself on the shitty excuse for a bed, the uncomfortable temperature of the place, being hungry, the crummy layout—consider yourself lucky if you get an actual room instead of a crumbling wall and three drawn curtains—the IV pokes, the hard X-Ray board, the tight squeezing blood pressure cuff, the staff that just wants to talk business, not make conversation, and still being in that place after seven or eight hours, patients nearly always reach a point of 'no more.'

They blow a gasket and refuse further movement, whether it's a repeating lab, a double check on their EKG, an additional type of imaging or consultation. They always reach a point of "Fuck this, I'm out." At which point the Nurse needs to divert their attention away from the four, five, maybe six or more other patients that all have steadily rising temperatures of their own to convince the patient that their best interest is to push forward because leaving could be detrimental to their health, possibly to the point of lifelong ailment or deterioration to death. So all that can really be said to someone who is inexperienced in regard to serious injury or illness and what it takes to get back to normalcy is fairly simple: it's complicated.

I need to take a quick couple paragraphs to explain that there are times where little to literally nothing looks out of place with the work-up. In times like these, Doctors will do what a coworker of mine once called 'Quilt Doctoring'. This is where the Physician will cast a wide net with the patient's work-up but in waves or baby steps (Note: A work-up is the series of tests ordered/performed by the medical team). They will order blood work, EKGs, and X-Ray images. They see what sticks and what doesn't. They are obtaining the entirety of the picture through patchwork. Also, the typical outcome from this is that nothing is found to explain the patient's complaint. The problem with this scenario is when you take into account all the minuscule things that try to throw roadblocks at a Nurse, returning to the same patient, giving the update that there is no new news and answering all the accompanying questions seriously defeats the Nurse's economy of movement. It's like the Nurse will have to walk three miles to accomplish what could've been accomplished in one.

It typically ends with the exact same type of patient response to the good news that no abnormalities were found and typically plays out something like this:

"There's nothing wrong!?"

This phrase is uttered with a "You've got to be kidding me!" tone as opposed to a "Oh, thank goodness!" tone so much more than I can currently find laughable.

Often, with these people, the Nurses want the work-up to find some minuscule thing, some minute abnormality with your workup. Why? Quite simple. It is easier to tell you how to fix something than to tell you that there is nothing wrong. In the neighborhood of three quarters of ER patients are discharged back to home, how many of these patients came in and were managed away from spiraling into an emergent scenario, I could not tell you but there are plenty of patients that come in sick but not dying. The ER figures out what is ailing them or their injuries are patched up enough to go home and continue the treatment plan at home or with regular visits to their primary care Doctor.

Those patients whose workups reveal nothing though? Telling these people that there is a small something on their X-Ray or that their potassium is on the low end, telling them something extremely minimal is so much easier than telling them that their workup is clean. Telling someone that their workup is clean is a half hour conversation that always leads to them proclaiming new symptoms. These patients love to wait until you are reviewing discharge paperwork before they announce that they aren't feeling well in some new way.

Now it is not only protocol but a standard of care that the Provider has a conversation with the patient prior to them being sent back home. And across the Emergency Rooms I have worked, this protocol has a strong batting average, it is really only in the face of a 'right here, right now' emergency where the Provider cannot step away from another patient that they don't review their work with a patient who is set to go home. These people gum up the working flow of the ER by not accepting the explanation given to them. The overarching truth of the situation is that the ER exists to identify and correct life threatening issues.

Sometimes, a patient will come in with a complaint and the ER offers no explanation as to why the person is feeling the way they are. It happens a lot. Here, the thing to know is that no immediate life threats were discovered. It doesn't necessarily mean nothing is wrong, it just means in the battery of testing the ER offers, nothing was found that is in the ER's realm to manage. It is entirely possible that whatever the ailment is could worsen to an "emergent situation" down the road, but the plan put forth by the ER here is to always follow up with a Primary Doctor, effectively handing off the plan to them. Usually, when patients return with a worsened condition that they were seen for, it was either a unique scenario where their issue worsened much quicker than anticipated or they never followed up with their Primary Doctor for further evaluation and monitoring.

Similarly, there are people who gum up the works after they refuse to believe the situation they are in is a simple one. A viral illness with a fever is a fantastic example. Various minor traumas are, too. Whenever a person comes into the ER for a fever and they are given Tylenol to break it, they are dumbfounded. They are typically angry. They hear "Tylenol" and fire back angrily, "Well, I could have done that at home!" The other end of the conversation is a wide-eyed RN thinking, "fuck yeah, you could have" while informing that Tylenol is the standard of care.

Which is, in the end, I guess one of *my* ultimate chief complaints: "You could have." You could have paid attention while driving instead of texting, you could have put down smoking years ago, you could have waited to watch that YouTube video until *after* slicing tomatoes with a sharp knife, and you could have just accepted the fact that as we get older our bodies break down . . . and injuries are more common if you fail to take care of yourself, exercise, and eat right. But you didn't err on the side of caution in any of things. So now we get to meet in person! There are, however, some prospective patients out there who understand that the emergency room isn't there to make them feel twenty years younger. It is to make sure they aren't going to die in the near future. I mentioned the 'turn your smartphone off and turn it back on again' situation at the very beginning. Here you go. Sleep on it.

PART 2: GATHERING INFORMATION

There is a reason hospitals contain more than just an Emergency Room. Each floor and department serves a purpose. The ER is the *initial* aspect of the hospital process as a whole for many patients no matter where they end up.

Some go home, some stay overnight, some make it their extended home for a period of time and some never leave. No matter where the eventual destination, where the ER begins, is triage. While the purpose of triage is to make rapid educated guesses as to who is more sick and who can wait a few minutes. The ER's purpose on the whole is to learn the severity of how sick or injured a person is, put a plan together, then move on. It isn't *meant* to be where patients stay for days on end like the sweet old lady had to. So, from the time a patient shows up, the team there is already thinking (in the back of their mind) about whether or not that person can go home versus a potentially longer hospital stay. The path to arriving at that decision is unique to each patient.

Sometimes the decision is obvious: if a person rolls through the ambulance bay doors with a backdrop of blue flashing ambulance lights and looking like their next stop is facing judgment in the afterlife (or whatever comes next) well then, I would place bets on that person not going home from the ER. Now, when someone comes through those ambulance bay doors, relying on a *different* person to keep blood pumping to their brain through CPR, instead of native heart function, the likelihood that they spend a certain amount of time in the ICU is high. Yes, truth can be stranger than fiction, but when things like that happen, the magic 8-ball is going to read, "OUTLOOK NOT SO GOOD".

And in times like these, when life hinges on swift medical action, there is a strong likelihood the ER staff will dive into a protocol. Protocols are designed for rapid movement, like muscle memory but for the entire department. Multiple things need to happen and if not at once, then in very rapid succession. Similar to the acronym for triaging sick patients—remember, ABC's?—protocol provides a checklist to manage very complex situations—it is a well-studied series of tasks that need to be completed, typically in a certain order and in the emergency room, with rapid timing.

The entire process is designed to eliminate the 'Put a Plan Together' aspect. "The Actual Plan" is predetermined and consists of a series of events needing to take place rapidly for those sick patients such as stroke, heart attack, or severe injury. The typical ER stay is an investigative process that sometimes takes hours to hash out. When someone's major organs are threatened, you don't have hours, you might not even have minutes. The goal in these scenarios is to stabilize —do their best to make sure the person isn't going to die in that room—and get the patient to the most appropriate place for longer term management.

All that business discussed above is the shit that makes internet videos for 15 minutes of fame or writes the script of TV Dramas. However, most of the time the situation's cause isn't staring you in the face and requires some information gathering to determine the answer. Medical shows would be much less entertaining if they showed 60 minutes of nothing but patients waiting with occasional updates.

The typical ER stay is a drawn out process and not a linear one at that.

This is because each person has their individual history without regard to the reason they are there and barring imminent death, you have to take the time to gather information first. Each has their own, unique story medically, surgically, socially, etc. Now, take the nearly endless amount of reasons a person can have for needing medical care, and toss in their various medical histories and the "next steps" aren't always so clear cut. Sometimes jumping into action without information will cause harm. Sometimes a situation is not an emergency per se but could progress that direction if not managed correctly.

The accumulated history of a person can add some serious roadblocks to their care. Take, for instance, someone who has experienced an allergic reaction to an antibiotic that, per protocol, is the most appropriate type of infection. The hospital team, depending on one's medical history, should pivot in order to help that person. In adults, their medical and social histories have a strong relationship. There are parts of their history such as types of heart failure, high blood pressure, obesity or obesity-related diabetes, kidney complications, liver complications, etc. that are married to decades of poor social and lifestyle habits. Decades of alcohol, smoking, eating poorly, inactivity, and other things that are unfortunately more difficult to remove from a person's life than such as irritants or carcinogens.

A couple questions to ponder: In the throes of experiencing a heart attack, how many adults make a vow to trade that greasy burger for a grilled chicken salad? Even if they *do* make the vow, how many act on it?

I don't want to dive into what putting a plan together for *children* looks like, not here anyway. I only want it to be said there is a far less likelihood, with children of medical or social history informing our next steps in the process. After years of working alongside healthcare workers, my belief is that many professionals struggle working with children as patients largely because of the "innocence" factor, and it's completely understandable—a secret that surfaces from their subconscious, which could be the result of their *own* child as a past patient or a situation where a child bore a striking resemblance to their own. But the realization of a sick child hits different because children possess an innocence and inherent desire to live—they haven't spent decades slowly killing themselves. Many adults have.

Putting a plan together gains traction once we gather information for a patient in their present state. The first step after triage and moving forward with a patient—unless there is a team of people slamming on their chest and pushing medications into their veins to keep them from crossing over into the afterlife—is ALWAYS an additional full set of vital signs and Physical Assessment. Sometimes a chief complaint will dictate the add-ons that need to happen to help a patient, but three things will certainly dictate the ancillary needs are a full set of vital signs, blood analysis, and a physical assessment.

From there, the team can look at the overall situation and determine if they need to obtain an X-Ray or CT Scan, which might lead the Provider to know or suspect that they will need to set a bone and splint it, or if they need to get cultures of a wound or swab a person's nose, etc. The nursing team is already thinking if they need to set up to assist the Provider for something like a pelvic exam, or if they need to start cleaning/irrigating a wound for sutures, or if they need to get an eye exam set up, place a urine catheter, etc.

Most often, the drafted plan needs to be updated or pivoted based on how things shake out from the means of gathering information.

VITAL SIGNS

Vital signs are a group of observable measurements obtained that reflect what a person's vital organs—heart, brain, lungs, etc.—are doing and "how" they are responding to whatever the patient is experiencing. Your vital signs are wildly important. They are a reflection of certain organs and have a normal operating range; the first set of these measurements are the baseline for a patient's stay and are a reference point for now only how effective or ineffective treatment interventions are.

A full set of vitals contains one's heart rate, blood pressure, respiratory rate with quality of breathing, oxygen saturation (which the staff typically calls the "oxygen level"), temperature, and the pain level that is also debatable as an additional vital sign. Pain is attached to nearly every reason a patient comes to the Emergency Room. I mean, pain is a means for our body to tell us that something is wrong. A lot needs to be said about pain because it is one of the absolute largest components of any emergency room throughout the United States . . . or world for that matter. If you are ever in an emergency room, put your ear to the wall and you can likely hear the painful wailing of someone less fortunate than you.

Now, a healthcare professional can sort of "determine" pain based on the objective measurements of other vital signs and where they are compared to normal ranges. Pain will cause your vitals to typically go up: faster heart rate, breathing, elevated blood pressure. Or if a patient is displaying something that is obviously painful. Think of how much it sucks to stub your toe—then consider stubbing your toe hard enough to cave it into the foot. That shit hurts.

Pain is difficult to quantify because it is, again, subjective. I mean, pain from a sore throat can suck but I'm guessing that pain from birthing a human sucks more. (Or so I've heard). The first time I encountered a patient with pancreatitis, I thought the guy was having a heart attack. No joke. But the next time I encountered pancreatitis, the guy was sitting there rubbing his belly describing discomfort like he ate a bad burrito—same diagnosis, very different presentations. So, while there are consistencies with injuries and illnesses, there is little consistency with the pain associated. This is why we ask patients to rate pain on a scale. A scale from zero to ten. Zero is typically a constant, but it is the opposite end that can just get ridiculous. There is a lot of room for interpretation. So yes, the pain scale is there but it is sort of like the Pluto of Vital Sign measurements.

There are actually multiple pain scales in use. The most common is pain rating from zero to ten that has two broad interpretations. For both, the zero end is pretty damn universal. Zero means no pain at all. It is the 10 part that gets ridiculous. Some healthcare providers will use 10 as the most amount of pain that the patient has ever felt in their life and compare their current pain to that. Then some will use 10 as the worst pain imaginable, which is just stupid for the simple reasoning that in this scale two different people are using their imagination—it also shines a light on how dumb some of the Nurses and Doctors can be as well. I mean, we're human, too.

After asking the patient how bad their pain is on the 0-10 with 10 being the worst imaginable and the patient rates their pain high, typically 10 for most instances. If the person asking doesn't believe the patient they will engage in a wasted time conversation comparing imaginations. For instance, the patient with abdominal pain will say it is a 10 out of 10 but not "appear" to be in 10 out of 10 pain. This will prompt the Nurse/Doctor to describe some of the dumbest shit. They will say, "So you're telling me that your pain is a 10? The WORST. Now, if a tiger came in here and breathed fire on you then chewed off your leg, that would be the same amount of pain you are having right now?"

Insert whatever fucking ridiculous scenario you want: Jason Voorhees chopping you up, Aliens filleting you alive . . . whatever. It is a waste of time to engage two people who are clearly not only on two different pages about pain.

The pain scale where the patient's current pain is compared to previous pains in their life is another use of the pain scale. This has the personal subjective history of patients and as mentioned, pain is your body's way of saying, "hey something fucked is going on right now, maybe get that looked at." But this scale is open to scrutiny from their history, if a person has never been in pain before well then there isn't much of a comparison. Science is now saying that emotional pain is in direct comparison with physical pain . . . let's just not open the door to that pain multiverse, okay?

Then there is an actual pain scale hung up on the wall. I really believe one that shows where we're at as a society—with zero to ten as they correspond to emoji faces! The zero emoji starts with big ole teeth and eyes popping out of a smiley face. As the numbers climb that smiling face slowly disappears, as three or four progresses, that smile is formed into a less curved smile and more of a concerned straight line. As the numbers escalate, the face goes from a trembling lip to "no more eye contact" emoji all the way to a streaking tears wailing face. Variations of this emoji scale exist, but they all have the same context of going from happy go lucky to inconsolable. This doesn't quite hit the mark either because a person could be in a tremendous amount of pain but think, "Well fuck, I am in a lot of pain but I'm not going to cry about it."

The pain scale that I like to use is based on the situation. I mean, it only seems appropriate to learn about and trend the person's pain for right there, right then. I mean, They aren't in the ER for a pain they experienced 12 years ago . . . despite how they may begin telling the story for their chief complaint. I will ask them basically 0 to 10 where 10 is that their current pain is so bad that focusing on anything else is a task. The middle ground numbers are variations of mild to severe pain but able to be distracted or able to rest without the pain disrupting things like conversations with family members, scrolling through social media, or watching TV, etc.

Basically, if you can complain about the ER decor, your pain isn't too awful.

Lastly, some people will go higher than 10. I will ask them the pain scale measurement and they will say 20. Well, if you are in pain that is not 'everyone on my social media needs to know about this' pain, you don't even think about being snarky. You answer 10. People that give the useless 15 out of 10- answers. Fuck them. The End.

Along with the patient's pain scale/tolerance, Nurses bring tools into the mix to further qualify a patient's vital signs. Plenty of cables, tubing, and devices . . . one of which is a stethoscope. You likely know it as the flimsy Y-shaped device hung around the necks of Doctors and Nurses. The device that sits in our ears and is typically worn backwards by actors in medical dramas. It gives us a smidge more information than we can detect without its help.

A standard stethoscope experience: I ask the patient for a couple deep breaths while I check out their lungs, they breathe in-and-out once before belting out in conversation, and through my end of the stethoscope device (which amplifies sound), their commentary comes through like turning on headphones you didn't realize had the volume on full blast. With most things, your heart and lungs are a marriage, if one is struggling, so shall the other. So, while I am recovering from an assault on my eardrums, I will take a quick listen to a patient's heart sounds as well. Realistically, it is pretty rare that any cardiac complications will be *heard*, cardiac complications will be picked up through other means like a detailed ECG called a 12-lead. My stethoscope might pick up some turbulent blood flow through your heart but overall, it is not going to differentiate a heart attack versus that burrito coming back for revenge. A detailed ECG is likely the most necessary piece of the puzzle in determining if your heart is struggling. With any chest pain complaints, a standard of care amongst hospitals is obtaining a 12-Lead ECG within 10 minutes. It is probably the most valuable tool used in determining life or death in real heart attack circumstances.

So, if you ever have a chest pain complaint and the staff starts throwing stickers all over your chest, arms, and legs, that is not the time to tell them how long of a day you have had and it has been hours since you've eaten last. The tracing that the machine displays is very sensitive to movement & each turn of the little squiggly line represents important information about various anatomical aspects of your heart and how it is beating. So do your best to mind the little things like how cold it is, or how thirsty you are for 1-2 minutes while we make sure you aren't going to be zippered up in a body bag in the near future.

I am hesitant to talk in detail about chest pain and the process because I have already heard from my patients or their family members more times than I would like that they 'know the secret' to getting seen in the ER quickly. They think they are clever in showing up and claiming chest pain so they don't have to wait in the lobby. Hopefully one day there will be criminal charges for this but hell, who knows. Assaulting hospital staff is a felony but that doesn't seem to stop people from throwing punches when they are told the ER isn't a gourmet sandwich shop (there is a lot to unpack there, I know, we'll get to it). In summary, the wait really sucks, we've communicated that but embellishing or outright lying about your chief complaint just to be seen sooner is an act of selfishness that could cost someone else their life.

Blood Pressure. Oh, Lord . . . blood pressure. The blood pressure cuff is that item that wraps around your arm and puts a squeeze on it. (We've seen all those fun machines at Wal-Mart that kinda look like a messed up fortune telling machine all over America). The higher your blood pressure is, the more pressure is exerted on your arm to obtain the measurement. The process of obtaining blood pressure typically takes roughly 30 seconds and in nearly every Emergency Room in the nation is taken by a machine that does it automatically. Like previous vital signs, this *should* be a simple process but gets muddied all the time because as soon as the cuff gets mildly tight people will raise their damn arm and scream at the thing (or the Nurse) like we are amputating their arm. Guess what that action does? It confuses the machine because the person is reacting so intensely it cannot obtain a proper measurement. The machine thinks it needs to pump a higher amount of pressure into the cuff. In the first Harry Potter movie, there's a pit the kids fall into called "Devil's Snare" which are tree vines that squeeze high school wizards tighter the more they move and struggle about. The way to get out is to remain still and just breathe. Same goes for us Muggles and blood pressure. Just relax.

Patients will typically ask me why it needs to be so tight. I have yet to find a clear, concise way to explain to them that I am not making up their blood pressure nor am I programming the machine to "unnecessary pain" mode. If your blood pressure is high, it is going to get tight . . . if your blood pressure is "normal", well then, you are the reason I don't like the subjective pain scale.

To round out putting a plan together necessitates a closer look at temperature. Temperature tells a lot of things. Your body is constantly trying to maintain its state of functioning within pretty tight parameters, all things considered, and your temperature is a reflection of the process. About the time you learn your ABCs, you naturally pick up on that if you are running a temperature—it is an indicator that your body is trying to fight off some nasty bug. There are other reasons for an elevated temperature, but let's keep it simple for now. The takeaway is that your body temperature has a range that is sustainable for living, just like all the other vital signs.

Similar to tracking other vital signs, Nurses will track your temperature as well—, and it's crucial to track with accuracy to know if an intervention is effective. In those crucial circumstances, tracking needs to occur at a person's core temperature. Think of when you microwave something. The outside feel isn't always an accurate representation of what is happening inside, which is why chefs will stab into a steak to know how "well done" it is . . . see where I am going with this? A core temperature is most accurately done by placing the thermometer probe inside a patient's butt. Sorry for the bad news.

To paint an entire picture of this Part in the book, we're gathering information—vitals such as heart rhythms, lung regularity, and blood pressure—while multiple things are happening at once. A Nurse might enact these procedures while asking you questions about your chief complaint. Multiple staff members—Nurses, CNAs, EMTs, ER Techs, Providers—might be involved in the process, too, if the place isn't running rampant. But a general rule is that the fewer people in the room, the less likely you are dangerously sick. Of course, no day is the same in the ER so don't panic if you ever find yourself, as a patient, in the ER while four staff members enter the room—it may have just been that way. Gathering information seems like quite the process, as all of this can get underway within the first minute or two after triage. It's all in prep for the Lab Work and Physical Assessment to commence.

LABS

IVs and labwork are additional tools used in the ER. A blood panel is standard for the vast majority of reasons people check into the ER. I mentioned earlier about how Star Trek medicine doesn't exist. This is typically where I need to have that conversation with people. Drawing blood for lab testing requires a needle poking through your skin to collect the red stuff into tubes and send it to the lab for testing depending on the purpose. Having anxiety over this is fine. Totally fine. As most people did not pencil "Emergency Room" into their schedule and plenty of people have a fear of needles. Got it. When it becomes difficult is when a patient tries to negotiate.

We lay out a plan to address the patient's needs (including the blood draw) and "Is that really necessary?" comes as a common response. The vast majority of the time, a blood draw *is* necessary. A patient's blood panel tells one hell of a story. It can reveal aspects of chronic and acute health complications. It can reveal how a person's body is handling systemic complications as well as bracket in on individualized organ function, and until Apple develops a watch that can break down blood components and chemistry, it's the method we'll use. The medical professional in me understands that education is the best thing available in nearly every situation—aside from elaborate griping, it is indeed a motivating factor behind writing this. So, I enjoy giving a quick education and holding a brief Q&A about the plan to help the patient. But the dark side of me just wants to say, "I'm not doing this for *MY* health. And yes, it is necessary."

Beyond collecting blood, an IV is one of if not the greatest tool in the Emergency Room. It is not an exaggeration to say that an IV is a lifesaving setup. Using an IV, immediate acting medications can be delivered to reduce pain or sedate, rehydrate, affect blood pressure to perfuse organs, etc. As noted above they assist in blood collection to detect abnormalities and are a key player in imaging that is used to detect injury.

If we cross paths and I am not at work, I will tell you that I am not a superstitious person, not even slightly. However, inside the walls of an Emergency Room, superstition reigns. There are not many instances where I will see myself as more skilled than another Nurse. However, when it comes to obtaining intravenous access (getting an IV), I am typically pretty damn good. I am nowhere near perfect but it is actually a skill I take pride in. Now, whenever the overall plan is discussed with a patient and the time for obtaining labs has come, as I am setting up to do so, it is not uncommon for the patient to remark "Are you good at this?"

As I said, with most patients, gaining IV access has become a mastered skill . . . so the "Are you good at this?" remark is the nursing equivalent of a restaurant customer responding with "How about a million dollars?" when the server asks if they would like anything else—followed by annoyed, awkward silence. Such a joke is overused and dumb. I don't have the vocabulary to tell you how overused and dumb it is so I'll just swear: it's equal parts unoriginal and fucking stupid. Let me tell you that their chances of things going well just took a nosedive. Maybe not "crash and burn into the Earth" bad, but they have fallen hard. If I had to try and explain why this is the way it is, the best I can come up with is either A) supernatural forces have reduced the likelihood or B) after that joke has filled the air for the 76th time that day alone, the Nurse attempting an IV is a little more dead inside.

With most modern emergency room procedures, obtaining a CT (Computed Tomography) Scan is a great likelihood. If undergoing a CT scan, patients often require a substance called "contrast dye" which is used to flush through a person's vascular system, permeate the person's bodily systems, highlight and 'contrast' (as shown on the scan) normal anatomy from abnormal. Accomplishing this correctly means the whole process needs to happen fast. The dye needs to be injected through an IV that not only is of a large enough caliber to handle the rush of fluids through it but it also needs to be in a vein that is large enough and stable enough to handle that flow as well.

This is why, when a patient shows up to the ER and the staff looks for a place to establish an IV, they typically look at the inside bend of a patient's arm. Typically, those veins are large enough and anchored into the arm well enough to withstand the power needed to deliver the contrast, allowing rapid flow to the body part that the Physician wants to focus on for their evaluation. Not everything is premeditated like this but when it comes to the overall evaluation, small steps can aid the process. Now, of course everyone's anatomy is different and a vein in that location might not be possible or as effective as a different spot. Flexibility is key—sometimes an IV along a person's forearm or, in absolutely necessary circumstances, their hand will simply have to do. I am unable to speak at great lengths on operating the CT Machine, I mean, hell that is an entire schooling in itself. But I do know that timing is important and the further away the IV is from the area that needs to be held to scrutiny, the more difficult the evaluation could be.

An important component in this "order of operations" is to know the results of the blood samples before conducting a certain type of imaging. The dye that is very useful in determining what is wrong with a patient is eliminated from the body by the kidneys. So, barring an extreme emergency or an absolute life or death situation, the results of blood samples will display how well a person's kidneys are functioning, translating to "If this patient gets contrast dye to better visualize their lungs, will it kill their kidneys in the process?" There are paths forward even for patients with suboptimal kidney function but all the members of the care team need to be informed. It helps add pieces to The Plan.

Superstition aside, there are several legitimate circumstances that add to the difficulty of gaining IV access—beginning with the fact that some people just do not have easy-to-find veins. If you line up 10 people who are nearly identical in all the major categories: age, sex, gender, race, lifestyle, etc. and have them hold their arms out . . . There is a great likelihood one or two of them will simply have *no* veins to find—no matter what. That shit happens. However, when it comes to medicine, you can't speak in terms of "IF *this*, THEN *that*." IF I throw a ball in the air, THEN it will come back down. That isn't how medicine works, that isn't how people work. In this field, we talk in terms of likelihood.

Nonmodifiable factors are things like injury and blood loss. Those will cause your veins to shrink down to prevent further issues. In some circumstances, being dehydrated is unavoidable. But conversely enough, it is also a controlled factor—volume loss in general is something that people can affect through their day-to-day activities. A person living off of energy drinks and caffeine is at a greater likelihood of being chronically dehydrated and having shriveled down little veins when compared to a person who consumes water regularly. Being frightened or nervous is going to cause those bad boys to disappear as well.

IF you eat a balanced diet and exercise regularly, THEN you are less likely to have health complications. Wouldn't we all love it if things were a guarantee? But they are obviously not. Bringing up anything in regards to physical features is ridiculously dicey territory, never is the purpose of ranting or explaining to shame in any way so do not take it as that when I tell you that there is a strong correlation between body habitus and difficulty establishing and maintaining an IV.

You can think of it in terms of hitting a target. Some complications shrink the target, some complications move the target, and some complications obscure the target. Then some do a combination of all three.

When I opened up talking about IVs a few paragraphs ago, I mentioned that one of the complications behind IVs is that some people simply don't have great veins. They are "difficult sticks" as we say. IVs are a skill that requires regular practice, and most people understand that Nurses are human and capable of making mistakes.

So, in summary, one of the things that increases the likelihood of teeing up a patient for a successful ER visit is establishing an effective IV.

Nurses need to own up to their shit, too. What is equally annoying is a Nurse who misses an IV, even if it looks like a beginner vein—one of those ones you can see from across the room. Nurses are expected to be professionals at their tasks, yes, but shit, even the people competing in the Olympics will botch a fundamental from time to time. It is all right when it happens. Owning up to your own shit and admitting error typically goes much further with patient rapport than saying some dumb shit like, "Oh, your vein rolled away." Or the healthcare favorite is, "I hit a valve." Saying these things makes the patient somehow feel like it is their fault when it isn't or that the situation was completely unavoidable. Neither are true.

IVs are a skill that requires regular practice. People understand . . . okay, MOST people understand that Nurses are human and capable of making mistakes. An area where professionals show distinction is acknowledging areas for improvement. It is in the same vein (wink wink) as saying, "The first step in fixing a problem is understanding that there is a problem."

Off-topic thing to say on the topic of IVs: consider a wild scenario like in the movies where someone is threatening to inject a syringe of air into a person's IV line to kill them. Unless that IV is about the size of their hand or the injection site is right to the victim's heart, the potential victim should tell whoever is making the threat to go right the fuck ahead. It takes *a lot* of air to do damage or kill someone. I'm not on the side of the fence that this is *healthy*, I'm just saying those scenes in movies hold no stakes. Every now and again while utilizing an IV, air bubbles will trickle down the tubing. They are harmless despite how much the medication pump protests. The IV pump saving a person's live by alarming to a line of tubing where the Nurse completely forgot to prime the fluid through the tubing is like that joke about how many terror attacks the TSA has prevented at the airport. I'm sure it has happened somewhere ... right? .... RIGHT?

All-in-all, I understand the initial fear, for some, about getting an IV. But even if "it hurts" a little on the front end, the pain will go away, and until then the benefit of having IV access is worth the pinch if it saves a life.

Thus far, we have talked about blood. However, not all labs are blood.

If you are contemplating going to the emergency room for literally anything potentially related to your belly region, you will need to provide a urine sample. There are multiple items a urine sample can tell the emergency team a lot about a complaint. At the very least it can rule out a couple things. A urine sample can reveal information on kidney health, if you have thyroid complications, diabetic complications, some neuro complications, pelvic trauma, or even complications of systemic trauma. It is incredibly useful.

I may take back my statement on vital signs being the easiest part of a patient's stay. Providing a urine sample should probably be the easiest thing one does at the ER. Take a piss and that's it. Well, that is close to it. The urine sample needs to be free of contaminants that live on your skin so really, the process is: piss a little then stop & clean your nasty self, then continue pissing into a cup. It is basically something you do multiple times a day with two added steps and yet when asked to in the ER to do so people act like we are asking them to carve out a pound of flesh.

"Oh, I just went before I got here." is the absolute most common phrase in response to asking for a urine sample. Which is fine, the plan at that point then pivots to other things like, see what shakes out in the bloodwork and get any sort of imaging done that has been ordered, give any medications, assess and reassess. But eventually . . . the Doctor is going to want that pee. I mentioned it before but for real, a urine sample tells a lot about the state of your health.

A certain amount of people are concerned with the hospital running a drug test with their urine. If you are unconscious or acting strange, then yes a urine drug screen will likely be ordered for the necessity of treating you as a patient. If a person is acting out of sorts and it is due to their belly full of Xanax, or Ativan, or Valium, or Klonopin because they had a particularly stressful week and needed additional help with their social anxiety, generalized anxiety, or panic disorder. I'm being harsh, as having an anxiety disorder would be miserable. But the take home message here is that there are prescribed medications that can be easily overdosed or there are illicit drugs that can absolutely mess you up. It shouldn't come as a shock to you that America (probably the world) has a prescription drug problem. Typically, one of the first interventions done for a person that is displaying what we call an "altered mental status" is in fact, to give the reversal agent for opioid medications. A urine sample isn't needed to do that but it will be needed to confirm.

Running a urine test to investigate other organ issues is way more common. It is actually quite regular. As mentioned a couple paragraphs ago it can reveal a lot about your health yet people feel like the ER has a pair of cops around the corner lying in wait and as soon as that result comes through positive for cannabinoids they will bust into the ER room with a ticket. Shit, the police don't even stick around after they drop off a wildly combative patient that had to be muscled in by three of them and two EMTs. They will give report to the Physician and myself like, "yeah we were called to this guy attempting to kick down his ex-girlfriend's door, he has been drinking since this morning, refused to breath for an alcohol level has been threatening to murder all of us the entire ride here, too. We thought he should have a Psych Eval and initiated the paperwork." The whole time the patient is in handcuffs glaring at me and interrupting the report with things like, "Fuck you guys!" while maintaining unblinking eye contact with me. This actually preludes a scenario where a urine drug test is absolutely needed. An Emergency Psychiatric Hold . . . we will save that fun for later or skip to Part 6 if you don't want to wait.

I digress.

One of the most dreadful scenarios for an ER Nurse is when the elderly check into the ER for "Altered Mental Status." For elderly *women*, specifically, this is a guaranteed encounter with a vagina that is on approach to the century mark. The old phrase 'Where the sun don't shine' is more like "The place where all but time has forgotten." It's like New York's undercity where maintenance hasn't been done since 1962. When elderly people seem to flip a switch and start behaving like they ran a hate group before retirement, one of the easier to root out causes is a urine infection. Women are especially susceptible to a urine infection simply because the plumbing is different. Not that it is impossible for males to get a urine infection, especially if they aren't snipped, but there is a hell of a lot more going on with the ecosystem between a female's legs than that of a male. I'd almost rather fight the drunk guy nightly.

This isn't as simple as peeing into a cup. Hell, there is a strong likelihood that an elderly person with "Altered Mental

Status" will be unable to follow directions anyway. At least with old men, when they get confused, the difficulty seems to be with getting them to keep their clothes on. But this urine sample needs to be clean for the Physician to treat it appropriately. This means a catheter. No, not an IV catheter. A urethral catheter. This means fighting through decades of skin stuck together and the smell that comes with it to find a small hole that, year after year, migrates farther and farther away from where it was originally located and thread a tube into it to drain out urine. All in the name of not having a urine sample contaminated by all the awful things that are living and growing on the outside of a person (hey, such a state is where we're all headed. In the end, gravity wins). Keep that aspect of the job description in mind the next time you haven't seen your Nurse for an hour. Also keep in mind that this situation is pretty much a once per shift ordeal for many ER Nurses.

Those are the moments I truly feel for anyone accompanying the craziest of patients—in this instance, Snot Lady's daughter. Nevertheless, part of a Nurse's job (whether someone is waving snot in your face or not) is to fight through the phlegm, maybe even collect it for lab testing, maybe put on an effort to conduct a Physical Assessment. and assess whether the patient can get out of dodge or stick around for a little while.

IMAGING

Imaging has become an essential part of figuring out what is wrong with a person. We'll certainly integrate how imaging helps the ER staff right around the corner, here, but just know the basics right here. Oddly enough, the first thing I am going to bring up is the ER Bed. Why the hell talk about the ER bed under the "imaging" header? Because the second most common complaint about being in the ER after the waiting is the bed. It sucks. It shatters all the hopes of things getting better after a patient has waited in the waiting room for 90 minutes. Initially, it is better than the long forgotten chairs that make up the petri dish that is the waiting room but after about, oh, 10 to 15 minutes, that bed in the ER room is going to feel closer to a prison cot than a sleep number.

The reason I am mentioning this is because in the ER patients need to be mobile and even on a good day most people are not very mobile. Now add in the additional pain, shortness of breath, dizziness, etc that accompanies why people are in the department. So, the bed needs to be light and mobile, after a few thousand patients this translates to worn down and rickety. But with a simple flip of a foot pedal to unlock the brakes on the wheels, a patient can be whisked away to X-Ray, CT, or wherever they need to go. At times, the imaging can come to the patient if it is a simple one-take X-Ray or an ultrasound, however, you can bet that the CT or MRI machines are permanently parked. And again, until the day Elon Musk invents Star Trek medicine and Physicians can focus imaging on individual body parts with a little holographic display in the room, off to them we go.

There is a lot of back and forth, two steps forward, one step back sort of a deal. Physicians don't like to irradiate people anymore than they need to so sometimes they will start with an X-Ray and if they don't see what they were hoping for, they move on to a CT. Sometimes, the Physician knows immediately that a CT will be needed—we talked about this with the IV situation not too long ago—if a family brings MeeMaw to the ER because she fell and she takes a 'blood thinner' pill for her aging heart, guess what? Straight to CT she is going. A CT is the current standard for identifying internal bleeding. Where this makes a Nurse's life a nightmare is when people preemptively throw a tizzy because of claustrophobia. Or their spinal column has endured five or six too many twisting, jerking motions and now a person cannot lay flat without 10 out of 10 pain.

Patients will sometimes require a mild dose of assistance to help with obtaining the correct image. Taking a patient to one of these machines is all for not if the patient is doing the 'fish out of water' thing while the radiation passes through them. The resulting image will be blurry and the task will need repeating. Sometimes, the patient to Physician stalemate of "I'm not doing that" vs "I need this to take care of you" places the Nursing staff squarely in the middle. Nurses already have half a dozen other patients needing their attention as they cry out in pain, throw up all over themselves, or simply throw a temper tantrum, none of us have time to play mobile negotiator and run through the human equivalent of Meerkat Manor like it's No Man's Land just to inch along the plan of care.

Outside of that, imaging techs are another great example of how RNs are the sandwiched profession in the ER. Keep an ear out if you are ever unfortunately in the department as a patient or with a patient. Most of the time as the representative from the imaging department leaves the room, the patient will ask for something and the response that can be heard all over the ER is, "I'll ask your Nurse."

PART 3: CARRYING OUT THE PLAN

There is no such thing as a pain free option. Hopefully I speak for ER Nurses across the country when I say that. For me, if I could summarize one of the largest challenges of accomplishing the job, "no pain free option" would be at the top of the list, edging out "no you cannot have anything to eat or drink until your scans are back".

Examples to the winning phrase include but are not limited to: the right kinds of cuts require cleaning and stitches, (which it isn't the stitches per se, it's getting to the stitches which requires numbing and if you doubt patients would choose shouting cuss words at staff and threatening violence over a couple of numbing injections you are dead wrong), broken bones need a little manipulation, bowel obstructions need a tube called an NG tube-tube threaded through a patient's nose into their belly, it sucks. Everything about an NG tube sucks from the insertion to the maintenance to the actual function which is to pull out all the contents in the stomach. In doing so, however, it gives the person's bowels time to heal by allowing them to rest—their own version of sleeping it off.

Anyway, the point is, nearly everything about being in the ER sucks. Hell, a good portion of the time, even just assessing a patient's chief complaint offers its own amount of discomfort. This part of the ER stay is crucial and also ties into various other components. Without beating on a dead horse, having a streamlined chief complaint determines where and how we assess our patients. If you come in with a laundry list of complaints, it creates disarray in formulating a plan. It immediately puts the RN and the patient on separate pages about what needs to be done and how to get there.

Performing the actual assessment is where the RN needs to maintain their "A Game". If it is fair to ask our patients to keep it simple with their chief complaint, it is fair to ask an RN to assess efficiently. Part of our job is to determine any outlier assessment findings and send the information to the ER Provider so they can have a more efficient (less time consuming) meeting with each patient. If an RN assesses appropriately and even saves the Physician five minutes, that translates into a lot of efficiency for over 100 patients a shift. That in turn decreases the amount of time it takes to put a plan together and get each patient on their way to their normal state—notice I didn't say back to health because ya know, ya'll some unhealthy people in general.

Relationships are give and take; here, the RN and patient relationship demonstrates this by asking the patient to keep it simple. We don't expect you to know exactly what is wrong so just say something general like, my shoulder hurts. Or my shoulder hurts when I raise it in front of me/off to the side, etc. We don't expect you to say things like, "my acromion process hurts" or "I think it's my transverse humeral ligament." Hell, that isn't even always an RN's position to take. Sometimes, you cannot even pinpoint it. Sometimes if you make a certain movement (shoulder example continued) the entire shoulder lights up with pain and you cannot determine exactly where. Our job is to define exactly which aspects are affected and how exactly through an assessment of the area. It requires some physical detective work and yeah, it can be painful but it is the ER version of carrying out the plan. Sort of a "think globally, act locally" to your overall health.

Ideally, the process goes: you tell us the general area, Nurses put the magnifying glass on it, and the Physician looks at the magnified area with a microscope. The plan comes together and the destination is plotted. Is it *THAT* simple? Almost never. Your body is made up of multiple systems, sharing living spaces and in constant back and forth communication. Assessments are uncomfortable but they are integral to identifying additional resources needed to further hammer out the plan. For instance . . .

FIRST STEPS

If your belly hurts, we've got to know which location and since your abdomen is a hollow area packed with guts, where you hurt isn't always where the pain originates. Nobody I have ever met has MRI vision so unfortunately, determining how to get our patients better means poking around a bit. It doesn't feel pleasant for the patient. The assessment of areas, in conjunction with blood results, can lead to detailed instructions on where to focus attention on a CT Scan or XRay. If your chest hurts, knowing if it hurts during certain parts of the breath cycle helps our overall assessment. As I mentioned, there are indeed times when an issue is a combination of things. Getting into a 50 mph wreck isn't going to focus all energy on one part of your body. Or a blood clot to your lungs is going to affect your heart and tissue oxygenation. Your body cannot cordon off problem areas like a submarine taking on water. Just not how it works.

Stitches and dislocated things are great examples of common ailments where a patient may have to endure a little pain to get to the other side of feeling better. You see, with lacerations, infection is a high possibility and the best defense is that whole prevention thing we mentioned early on. The sooner lacerations are cleaned out properly, the better chances someone has against complications related to healing and infection. This means Nurses often address an area that is already injured. To save the patient undue pain and grief, we use an injectable medication to numb the area. This has long-term effects but still, as you guessed it, it is painful at first. Patients fighting this initial series of injections is quite common.

Similarly, in order to reduce pain, promote proper healing and straight up put you back together again, a dislocated joint will need manipulation by the Doctor to realign a part into its normal position known as its "anatomical position." Sure, in preparation of the process, pain medication can be administered but it is still no picnic. If something is very far outside of its anatomical position, it may even warrant strong medication to put a person into a moderate sleep to accomplish the goal. Yes, the process of realigning something is anywhere from uncomfortable to outright painful, but this is a great example of the end justifying the means. Proper alignment of a broken bone in itself is a great analgesic not only in the moment but with long-term pain through healing and rehabilitation success.

Every time I go into a patient's room to follow up on how they are doing and they are waiting to tell me off because it has been an hour since I have seen them, I want to tell them exactly the scenarios you just read. "Well, you see I would have been here earlier but I had a patient with a laceration that was refusing the numbing medicine because they are afraid of needles." or "I had to calm down the guy across the hall for an hour because apparently he would have rather dealt with his broken arm by holding onto it instead of putting on a splint.

Hospitals frown on that sort of honesty though. The Charge Nurse (like, the Boss Nurse for the shift) quite literally has to pass down from management in the pre shift huddle to not say things like how busy you are to patients. How are Nursing and Stripping similar? Both professions are always to appear available. The idea is not to dissuade patients from asking for help—really not an issue for 9 out of 10 but sure. There are some modest people that "don't want to be a bother" The overwhelming majority, though? The hospital upper echelons would much prefer the Nurses take shit from their patients with a smile on their face over honesty.

Your body's natural stance on pain is to veer from the path that puts you in a painful position—it's our caveman instinct. Unfortunately, Nurses battle having to keep people cooperative with the plan to endure some pain even if it means literal life and death. I had a patient once who had been playing a game of recreational hockey and took an ice skating blade to the front of his wrist. You have two arteries that run down your arm along the sides and end in a network of little arteries that provide your hands with blood. This guy sliced completely through one of them and halfway through the other. Blood everywhere.

Typically, managing a large bleed involves a lot of pressure to slow or stop blood from exiting one's body. The pressure assists the body's own defense mechanisms by allowing the clotting factors in blood to patch up things. Arteries push blood through the body with a tremendous amount of force so any attempt the body makes at forming a clot to naturally stop the bleeding just gets blown away. In a situation like this, the required means of managing the bleed are exceptional.

To keep this hockey player's blood inside his body (instead of on the walls and floor) we used a specialized blood pressure cuff around the guy's forearm. This device has the capability of *holding* pressure instead of taking a measurement while it deflates. When enough pressure is used to cut off blood flow, the intervention is called a tourniquet. In this instance, a tourniquet was definitely required, and we inflated the cuff until the bleeding stopped before holding the pressure in place. Those normal means of stopping bleeding with direct pressure, elevation, and a hell of a lot more time than this guy had, are only effective once the force of all that blood has drastically slowed down . . . meaning the dude would have learned what happens after we die if we tried those means.

Also, in this situation all roads lead to a specialty Doctor—a vascular surgeon. An emergency room Doctor might be able to toss in a stitch or 20 to stop the guy from bleeding to death, but the answer is surgery to repair the arteries properly. And in these situations, vascular surgeons move fast. This guy went from ambulance bay doors to the surgical suite in about

PART 3: CARRYING OUT THE PLAN

45 minutes, which may seem like a long time to some, but is like warp speed in terms of surgical set-up and procedure.

Bloody Wayne Gretzky was just so impressed and grateful for the coordination and swift action! He smiled from ear-to-ear as healthcare professionals arrived and whisked him away to surgery!

Not quite . . .

Remember the Devil's Snare from the putting a plan together section? It is uncomfortable and it hurts. The injury itself hurts. There was no shortage of legitimate sources for pain. Unfortunately, this was one of those scenarios where no amount of medication was going to eliminate it all combined with the ugly truth that there was no pain free option to keep him from the clutches of death. This guy had a much better visual to teach him why the cuff needed to be on tight than I could ever put into words; he literally watched his own blood spray 10 feet across the ice at the pond as well as turn crisp white towels a gleaming crimson within seconds and *still* groaned about the cuff being too tight. The first thing he said to the vascular surgeon was, "Please take this thing off of me, the Nurse won't do it."

What I am getting at is that assessing patients can be a lot like those memes of a flowchart: does it move? [Yes/No] Should it [Yes/No] Is the person's blood going around and around or around and out? And while the ER is not intentionally a torture chamber, part of the process of narrowing down what is wrong with a person is if it can be replicated or not . . . if it has *timing* or not. The best Nurses and Doctors are also educators. They should tell you what they are doing and what to expect before they do it. However, sometimes the immediacy of the situation doesn't allow for a well-structured lecture. As a patient, it can be frustrating, and is like learning the dance as you go except with life or death consequences.

In the instance of certain emergencies, hospitals are recognized by how swiftly they move. For example, with a patient experiencing a heart attack—one of the veins of the heart is clogged and the tissue is dying. The only means of saving a person's heart is to remove the clog. The national standard is to have that happen within 90 minutes . . . with the kicker being from the beginning of the symptoms. So, if the paramedics come to your house to investigate chest pain, and discover on their EKG that a person is having a heart attack, they have 90 minutes (minus the amount of time since the heart attack) to give that person the best possible chance at surviving.

From the outside looking in, it can leave your head spinning, even with staff members keeping you informed along the way. There are multiple people looking, listening, assessing, starting IV's, hooking up machines, and giving medications. There's also plenty of questions and moving as it is all happening. Information like that is difficult to process at any pace when it is contending with worrying about the outcome of someone you care about.

When dealing with brain issues or complications, the national standard is 60 minutes (maximum) before death. It is insane to think about how the plan for a person's night could be to make dinner and watch Netflix, but by the time that show ends, the food is sitting out, cold and uneaten while the person who made it is in the hospital having a device threaded into their heart or brain to keep them from not only from dying but to also hopefully have some semblance of their quality of life saved.

RED TAPE

The ER is full of contradictions. Sometimes the scenario is a well rehearsed protocol like those traumas, strokes, heart attacks, etc. Sometimes, even with a general complaint there is a glaring piece of the assessment process that formulates the plan. However, a large amount of the daily ER function is when there isn't.

Sometimes, the destination isn't simple math like "broken bone, fix bone." Remember the term "Quilt Doctoring." Another term we use is "Nickel and Diming." This is where the Physician will cast a wide net with the patient's workup—they will order blood work, EKGs, X-Ray images—they see what sticks and what doesn't, then adjust the workup from there. It can be unbelievably frustrating on two fronts: 1) you really want to know what the heck is going on and provide answers and 2) as a Nurse you get really damn sick and tired of going back into your patient's room 20 times without a good direction on where things are going.

There is an aspect of medicine that promises the public: Physicians will only order necessary testing and treatment. But people also go bananas if they are left hanging, so Physicians sometimes work extensively to give them anything to work with. Especially if, for whatever reason, they have a gut feeling that something *is* indeed wrong. It is not uncommon for Doctors to ask patients to stay a night in the hospital just for observation. Hopefully, they have a boring night away from home, but in the event that whatever is ailing them has yet to fully present itself, it is better the patient stay in the immediate vicinity of tools/expertise necessary should the issue return. These situations typically come with a regular joke about how Nurses don't deal with money, too, as there is usually a joke about "racking up the bill" in air.

The truth there is that yes, hospitals are A-holes when it comes to billing. They typically charge up to 10 times what something should cost because they are preemptively entering the payment negotiations. Another truth is that the Nurse has literally zero to do with that but yet patients will resist the plan in an attempt to soften the blow of the bottom line.

Then there are Doctors, typically younger ones, that practice Chicken Little Medicine. I probably don't have to tell you what that means, but I will: they act like the sky is falling with every patient. I can appreciate thoroughness but when Physicians do this, it isn't being thorough, but it also isn't malice. The Doctor either just has that intuitive feeling that something is wrong or they haven't developed ER intuition and are checking, double checking, triple checking ... you get it. It does, however, create a backlog with every patient that comes in. Part of being a Nurse is to "assess" the providers you work with, too. Getting a feel for which Doctors, NPs, PAs, will order an entire smattering of tests will save a Nurse a lot of stress. The Nurse can know to draw an additional vial of blood for tacked-on testing. Or prepare the patient ahead of time by letting them know that the night will involve a lot of updates on things.

I've mentioned numerous times how people don't act like the ER is the ER. They act like it is a mall, a one stop shop, a day out on the town with a friend. They can get lunch, a massage, a nap, maybe some snacks later, oh and if there is time, they can get that 10-out-of-10 pain checked out. OR, maybe get that ugly thing that has been going on for a month and a half that you think is cancer check out at 2am.

For example, I once had a mother come into the ER at three in the morning with a wadded up tissue of snot. Yes, snot. She was utterly convinced that her daughter was coughing up the lining of her throat, and I could just not convince her that it was phlegm. I tried once or twice to describe upper respiratory signs and symptoms to a person who was plenty old enough to have had one or two herself but she was too busy literally unfolding the phlegm soaked tissues in my face as if to change my mind. I was more than happy to offer to collect it in a specimen container in the impossible event that the Physician thought it was less run of the mill phlegm and more cancerous tissue.

Such instances lead to an unfortunately common ER phenomena: "You're a *Nurse*, you don't know shit." Were those Snot Lady's exact words? No. But there are others who have expressed the sentiment in so many words. This "extremist" mindset from patients is rare but possible on any given shift. I will update a patient with the Plan We've Put Together on moving forward accordingly, and sometimes get an "I'd like to hear what the *Doctor* thinks" in response. Sometimes I don't care, like in the case of Snot Lady, as she didn't want to hear about a plan from "Just a Nurse" (She *did* say that). As a Nurse, you must let those words roll off the duck's back and let a Provider deal with that phlegm. Not your problem anymore.

Remember that the ER is just the tip of the iceberg. It is not the place to stay indefinitely. This seems like the utmost "well duh" thing to say at this point but also remember how I mentioned that the ER is a full time contradiction as well.

There is usually at least one patient a night that leaves an ER Nurse in a blank stare thinking, "what the actual fu ..." when they inform the previously 10 out of 10 pain patient that the Doctor would like to keep them in the hospital and the patient throws a fit about it, questioning how necessary it is.

Whenever the patient is milliseconds away from transport from the ER to wherever they will be staying in the hospital, a myriad of complaints will arise. Remember that primary care Doctor that nobody wants to bring into the loop? They are the ones to ask about your thyroid at an appointment, not the person with RN behind their name instead of MD. And most certainly not when you have been sitting in the Emergency Room for several hours getting your nausea under control should you bring up your concern for your LDLs.

Sometimes the plan has been pre-formulated. If a person comes to the ER with a complaint involving their major organs such as a neurological or cardiac complaint, there is a strong chance they are going to stay in the hospital at least overnight. Turn that strong likelihood into a guarantee if there is anything at all out of perfect alignment with the workup. For instance, with chest pain, even if everything lines up wonderfully, the effects of a cardiac event lying in wait are also very slow to reveal themselves. When under stress, your heart muscles will "leak" out certain proteins that are used as markers for dangerous cardiac events. It is sort of like sending out distress signals. The issue here is that the proteins take quite a long time to detect a difference (roughly six hours) and obviously then, an even longer time to develop a trend. So, anyone at or past middle age with a complaint of chest pain, the plan is already laid out for you and it isn't a quick turnaround.

PART 3: CARRYING OUT THE PLAN

Patients getting admitted into the hospital have several communicating pieces and I will tell you that the Nurses have maybe 10% to do with it overall and zero to do with it until the admission is finalized. It is all dependent on the capabilities of the hospital, the Physicians available – if there is a specialist involved, if the working group of Doctors admitting already have a full load of patients, taking on more might not be in the best interest of the patient.

Basically, a version of the following is what takes place:

1) It is determined through the ER workup that a person needs to come into the hospital.

2) The ER Physician gives notification of the patient's needs to the Unit Clerk who then gives the notification to the House Supervisor – basically the hospital's all seeing Eye of Mordor, they are the manager of managers that Karen dreams of speaking to.

3) The House Supervisor reviews if the hospital has availability appropriate for the patient's needs.

4) The ER Physician is not going to oversee the patient's care outside of the ER, so part of determining a patient's needs is searching for a Doctor in the field of the patient's needs & seeing if there is room in their Inn.

5) Next, when the admitting Physician gets involved and has a conversation with the ER Physician. They discuss the condition of the patient and if the Doctor that will be taking the handoff wants more information it can mean additional testing in the ER … so be prepared for more to be done there. Which may not seem like movement out of the ER but it is.

6) If everything works out swimmingly the receiving Physician's nursing staff is notified and the Charge Nurse on that ward then determines if their staff member is safe to take on another patient—sometimes more bodies need to be called in before the patient can be sent to their new location.

7) Once a receiving RN is assigned, they need to get up to speed on the patient they will be getting. This means a conversation known as 'report' on the patient by the RN that has been with the patient. Finding the time to do that can at times be tricky if either or both RNs are fully loaded with tasks.

Really, what you should take away from all of that is that first, the shit takes time. If things go smoothly it takes 30-45 minutes. And that is a SMOOTH admit a.k.a. vast MINORITY of admits. Typically I tell my patients to be prepared for an hour, give or take. The second thing is that through the whole process where do you see the Emergency Room Nurse involved? The very end for the Nurse to Nurse report, and there will be a quick thing or two about report to come.

There are things that I would like to relay about the plan for patients in the ER and one is that the plan isn't so much of a movement forward as it is like a pinball getting bounced around inside the machine. If reading through this thus far feels like trying to keep track of that pinball, it is partly because that is not too far off from how a Nurse feels every shift. Sometimes, carrying out a plan flawlessly will still have faulty results. There is a certain type of ugly "CYA" that I'm sure is a large part of the world we live in but in healthcare it is unreal. Just like patients will forget, it is almost like the system itself will forget that the path forward can be two steps forward, one step back. When that happens, it is impressive the lengths people will go to separate themselves from things that happened.

For instance, a patient being admitted into the hospital to monitor their cardiac enzymes for a subtle heart attack once decided to wait through the entire ER stay and literally on the transfer to the telemetry floor (cardiac monitoring), told me that he really needed to pee. Now, I figured he was like most normal human beings and was simply telling me that he needed to pee. Obviously, being pushed through hospital hallways while connected to a monitor and all the cords that come with that as well as having medications infused to protect his heart is not the setup for relieving yourself. I learned that night how long five minutes can be when a full grown adult is yelling at you every 20 seconds about how he has to pee.

On arrival to the room where he would be staying, he did what I have now come to expect people to do but at the time wouldn't have ever crossed my mind. He leapt out of the bed and began making his way to the bathroom. All his cardiac monitoring, oxygen monitoring, IV tubing became a total mess and nearly all of it became disconnected ... to include one of his two IV's. This guy put emptying his bladder before saving his heart. A rapid decision was made to intentionally disconnect the medication infusing to save his other IV. The receiving Nurse was notified of the recent events and informed of the silver lining that he had one remaining IV.

The trip back to the ER was barely long enough to cool down my anger with the patient but the ER doesn't wait. Time to get back to work. However, in this particular instance, I was pulled aside by the Charge RN as soon as I returned the empty bed covered in a tangle of monitor cables and asked to confirm if I had disconnected the medication that was infusing. I confirmed the statement but added that it was to save a longer delay because the patient was unable to be reasoned with and was unwilling to wait another couple of minutes to safely get to the toilet.

The lesson here is that in healthcare, people would rather go to the corners of the Earth to say "this wasn't my fault" as opposed to simply making note of where the plan veered off path and course correcting. The Charge RN that night informed me that the Nurse reported me not only to my department but to the Cardiologist who was assuming care of the patient. If that isn't ridiculous enough, the Cardiologist himself even felt the need to call down to the department hours later to get the offending Nurse on the phone and "educate" on the importance of not having a break in the medication infusing. The medication by the way, was a medication called Heparin, which has a half-life of roughly 60 to 90 minutes—meaning that it takes almost an hour and a half for the effective amount of the medication to be reduced in half. A bit much but hey, the point is the guy had a tight window of up to 90 minutes to pee.

There is also this peculiar ... almost paradigm ... where the opposite happens, it's absolutely wild. If there is a nightmare scenario and things workout swimmingly – or close to it; if there is a favorable out come – people will transform into a creature so chatty that a pack of gossipy grandmothers after church would look like a fucking silent auction.

They will insert themselves into the situation and tell anyone. For instance, if you work in an emergency room long enough you will eventually encounter the nightmare scenario of nightmare scenarios: infant arrest. It is an indescribably tense time. Typically, though you see the best in people come out, in the limited times I have been involved with it, the most common voice you hear is the Physician's. You will hear other voices that repeat back orders to the Physician for effective closed loop communication, but really, it is a quiet time where minutes seem like hours. Until it is over.

Then every pair of scrubs walking around wants to tell you their perspective.

"Holy shit! I was just walking out of my other patient's room when I saw [insert name] run by holding what looked like a lifeless baby! I just high tailed it after them and fucking blah blah blah!"

"Oh my God! I was getting a line while another Nurse was setting up the warmer and blah blah blah!"

The whole time you are sitting there like, "yeah, I was fucking there, bruh."

I tend to keep my words to myself in those situations though because that's how people cope and I do understand coping to my core. Even when the plan gets carried out to near perfection or even things simply just go right in high tension scenarios, Nurses still have this issue where you replay them in your mind to nitpick what could have gone better. At least I haven't had to witness any Nurses posting choreographed dances to TikTok. My initial reaction to seeing those situations is, "when the hell did you find the time?"

Outside of the small five bed ERs out in BFE, nearly every Emergency Department is full to the brim with patients. When the holy hell do these social media Nurses find the time to make those damn things? Plus, they make the profession look like attention seeking fools, if anything they lend a helping hand to every management that has suggested bullshit recognition like "Fastest Urine Collection Time" trophies or just having pizza parties in general.

Sigh

There is so much that can get in the way of actually "carrying out the plan" that it's a wonder the plan ever comes to fruition in the first place. The point is, there *is* a lot of red tape involved in the ER experience but there are *also* a lot of hardworking people with (proverbial) scissors to cut through said red tape and get the job done. There is too much at stake to fret about tape in the moment, as the only thing that really matters is "how are we going to execute this plan?" That's the question that fuels any ER staff, and how they communicate the *answers* to that question is how the chief complaint actually gets addressed and taken care of.

PART 4: COMMUNICATION STANDARDS

We'll keep shining a light on what happens when you get a bunch of humans in the same building, trying to fix our flailing and failing bodies. The good, the bad, and the jackassery . . . none of it is off limits when this phenomena is at hand. Combine the fact that yes, there are standards of care when it comes to treating patients, there are also minuscule details in how certain providers prefer to handle managing their patients.

Half of a Nurse's job is the psychiatry of figuring out how certain providers work and the best way to work with them. It is always centered around job proficiency and advocating for patients. A simple truth of the ER is that when working to help a patient, approaching two Physicians in the same manner could yield dramatically different results. If, for instance, a patient would really appreciate having some more pain medication. As an RN, informing two different Physicians with the same approach could yield responses on opposing ends of the spectrum from "thanks for the update,

I'll order more" all the way to "are you serious with this shit right now, leave me alone."

As a new and young Nurse, I was repeatedly baffled at how difficult the most standard communication could become. Looking back, I shouldn't have been—after all, this is the same country that is so divided on simple observations like the color of a goddamn dress that it makes national headlines.

If my book goes anywhere, I will likely have a bountiful amount of responses to the contrary with the following but most of the time (in my experience) interactions between Nurses and Physicians are strictly professional. It isn't all Grey's Anatomy where conversation is littered with, "What are you doing Saturday night?" Experienced Nurses learn to speak on topic, clearly, and concisely. The nursing field summarizes in-hospital communication according to another acronym, SBAR. The letters stand for *Situation, Background, Assessment, and Recommendation*. There is also the importance of notifying the Provider of pertinent changes.

For instance, if I had a patient that was experiencing respiratory distress, things would move along much faster if I approached the Physician with the following method of communication:

- **Situation**: The details around the reason they are in the ER. Essentially, this is the aforementioned "chief complaint" but now comprises information gathered through triage, Questioning, and so forth. *Disclaimer: In the event of a respiratory patient (ever-increasing in a post-2020 world), Practitioners SHOULD see you shortly, unless a good long nap restores you back to full, restorative breathing.*

- **Background**: Depending on the situation or chief complaint itself, Nurses converse with the Physician and give details such as the person's age, when the problem began and events surrounding the chief complaint such as activity, physical surroundings, and history of previous incidents. Again, all of this is a result of gathering Information, putting a plan together, etc. Let's continue with an example of a respiratory patient.

- **Assessment**: Assessment is critical, as you cannot simply approach a Physician and say "They can't breathe!" That helps absolutely nobody. Now, if a Nurse takes a fast listen and determines air is or is not entering a patient's lungs (and how far down or on both sides), and relays to the Physician an oxygen saturation and level of discomfort the patient is in, the Physician and be scheming and possibly placing orders on their way to see the patient. If the situation is critical enough, yes, the doc will be at the bedside and an RN worth their salt would have notified a respiratory therapist already.

- **Recommendation**: Providing a recommendation cannot happen without the previous steps in place. A Nurse cannot approach a Physician and say, "Uh, this person can't breathe, and they look like shit, I think we should do something about it." Based on the information gathered in the assessment phase, a Nurse can simply say the patient is critical enough to warrant the Physician at bedside. Sometimes, if it is not that critical you can give a recommendation—such as a breathing treatment with long-acting steroids to follow.

Now, with the major players that keep anyone alive—brain, heart, lungs—it is absolutely understandable the Doctor would want to be physically present with the patient. And with SBAR guiding the way, it certainly changes communication (and outcomes) according to the situation. Perhaps a Nurse is informing the patient's Doctor on the situation of a procedure or medication given. The outcome would then become something different.

Now, not every Physician responds to this type of communication equally. Sometimes a Nurse will ask a Doc for a medication change and they'll blow a few gaskets at how the Nurse would make such a recommendation. But that's never happened to me, of course (The biggest of JK's). An experienced Nurse knows that nursing is part poker-player in that you have to play the scenario out three to five steps ahead. For instance, with the Doc who did in fact rebuke *me* for a medication change, communication in that situation could have resembled the following:

"Excuse me, Dr. [Name Redacted]. I need to update you on your gallbladder patient. They are still in pain despite the medications you wrote, and I've given the medications ample opportunity to control her pain but they are not having the desired effect. Here are their most current vital signs. What would you like to do next?"

Again, there is a chance he still would have been a dick about it, BUT there is a class of Physician that responds favorably to feeding one's ego and a Nurse putting *theirs* aside to stoke a Doc's internal fire—it's all a common route taken to help any given patient. Most Physicians simply trust you based on how much time you have or haven't spent together. If they know you to be a reasonable RN, and you don't come to them with every little squabble, they are greatly inclined to respect your recommendation.

But going back to the whole humans in the hospital thing, jackassery included, we all know Physicians are people, too, so there is ALWAYS a chance the Physician will just flat out suck. But who knows . . . maybe Dr. [Name Redacted] is out there somewhere writing his own book about how Nurses who try to change a Doctor's medication procedures should have gone to medical school, that they flat out suck, or both. To each his own.

One of the takeaways is that when things don't go as foreseen by the patient, it isn't for a Nurse's lack of effort. Shit, blaming the decades of overly prescribed narcotic pain medications is probably a good place to start. In the ER, it will get you nowhere but it is still a better place to focus anger at hesitancy in pain management than at the Nurse. Sifting through the waves of people that claim an obscure 10 out of 10 abdominal pain in an attempt to get a drop of Dilaudid but will settle for a turkey sandwich, there is indeed people in impressive amounts of legitimate pain (I can personally attest) and it sucks that they deal with pain longer than they should but it is also true that a few million bad apples are spoiling the bunch. Physicians are now entering the medical field wearing their white coats like shiny suits of armor, standing ready to combat the opioid epidemic and I'm all for it. Hospitals have literal full scale training programs on alternatives for pain management. So if you are coming into the ER from a patient's perspective, know that the Vegas odds of pain management being a combination of non-opioid meds like Tylenol and physical modalities like ice and elevation are high. From a nursing standpoint, effective and accurate assessment, evaluation, reevaluation, and communication with the provider is imperative fuel that drives the plan.

The *main* point here is that, when done well, SBAR is a quality reminder throughout the ER process and, if you think about it, life in general. What's your current Situation? What

Background info do you have to take the next best step? How do you Assess what that next step is? And then make a Recommendation accordingly—either to yourself or to someone alongside you. They say that hypertension is the silent killer but any Nurse that works tirelessly to advocate for their patients, just to hit brick walls from the provider and then return to a room full of angry family members because "nothing is getting done" can attest to having the roaring ER sounds drowned out by the rush of angered blood pumping forcefully through their ears.

There are indeed nights where the ER looks like the total chaos depicted in medical dramas. It is indeed a pretty incredible place. There can be a room with three Nurses, two Techs, and one Doctor all actively engaged in saving a person's life that very minute and the next door down have an antic mother ready to shove her daughter's snot in your face while two hallways over there is a patient refusing to take the medication the Doctor wrote because the Nurse didn't put enough ice in their water. You will have nights where you have six patients to manage all at once needing everything from a simple medication to be given, a wound to be cleaned, to a procedure that needs to be set up to correct a person's irregular heartbeat, while another person is throwing up relentlessly, and finally you have an old person (who is weak on a normal day) even weaker now because they are sick and trying to get out of bed for the 11th time in three hours.

Even slight miscommunications for any given reason can cause delays or hiccups in patient care, which is most detrimental to the patient, yes, but also reverberates to other patients simply by mismanagement of time and resources. At a busy enough ER, inserting chest tubes is common practice.

PART 4: COMMUNICATION STANDARDS

They are used in situations where fluid or air is collecting within a person's chest cavity, which in itself is problematic but becomes immediately life-threatening if the substance builds up too much and impedes the functional ability of the lung(s) or eventually even the heart if it gets too drastic. To fix the issue, the Doctor will cut through the side of a person's chest, insert a tube to act as a drain and restore the balance. The drain tubing is attached to a collection container that is the Nurse's responsibility to monitor and manage.

The nursing team can set up for one within just a couple minutes while imaging confirms what the Physician needs to do. From start to finish this can be accomplished in 10 minutes. Now, medical equipment is just like any other consumer good and has competing companies make any product. One particular patient, a surgeon was consulted to place the chest tube and told the Nurse to set up for a "Pleur-Evac." A PleurEvac is the collection container that the Nurse would manage after the chest tube insertion. The problem being that the ER used collection systems called "Atriums." Literally, they perform the same task, just have minor differences in appearance.

Confused, the RN confirmed the request from the surgeon who, giving one of those smiles that doesn't quite match the look the eyes above it are displaying, responded with a cold, "PleurEvac." That poor Nurse speed walked from RN to RN asking where those specific containers were kept. Nobody knew, The Charge RN didn't know, the House Supervisor was notified to check with Surgery to see if they had one because the ER certainly did not. Half an hour went by and yes, the surgeon was pissed by now. The RN found the surgeon at a work station he had claimed to tell him that the hunt was still on.

That disregard for others by sitting anywhere is a thing all in itself, too. Specialty Doctors will show up and not a fuck who has been at a work station all night. Even though they have designated "doc boxes," whatever computer they choose is theirs as long as they are in the ER.

Anyway, the response to the news was, "I don't understand what the deal is here, it's not like we don't do these things several times a week." Upon hearing the rising tension, a different provider who regularly works in the ER stepped in on the conversation and informed the RN that an Atrium is what the other surgeon was indeed looking for. The real issue here is that the patient was delayed by more than half an hour because of two people using different brand names to describe the same thing. In a trauma bay, it's not the same as a muggy restaurant patio in the South where the wait staff asks you if you want a Coke.

Communication structure may have a place that is generally followed but the generational speak of pronouncing things slightly different or using a medication's (one of many) brand names over the drug name plays a part pretty regularly. This form of "to-may-toe" vs "to-mah-toe" speech doesn't always trip up the Nurse's night and delay patient care quite like that Atrium vs PleurEvac fiasco. It is typically a pretty decent laugh like, "haha you old man, you called the Nitro drip, Tridil. People haven't done that since before I was born," then we all move on.

SHADES OF GRAY

Working side-by-side with practitioners in the ER was best described to me by a Physician. She was a newer doc. Not only new to the ED but new to being a full-time Doctor;

however, had already shown herself to be quite capable and ridiculously personable. She didn't have a tremendous poker face but didn't exactly wear her heart on her sleeve. She showed the appropriate amount of stress for the situation. In the short time we worked together, she showed herself to be quite self aware.

The following quote occurred post-procedure on a patient for which she was the assigned doc and I was the assigned Nurse.

The patient presented the ED with an abdominal hernia that had worsened. A hernia is a weakened area of muscle in the (typically lower) abdominal wall which can result in an outpouching or protrusion of the deeper structures such as fat or even your bowels—gross, right!? So the treatment for this can be mild to severe depending on how new and how disgusting—professionally termed "Type" or "Severity"—the hernia is. This person had a pretty decently sized hernia in their lower abdomen, so the Physician determined the appropriate treatment would be to try to reduce the hernia. This means to try and push it back in. When a body part is out of place and you get paid an assload of money to make it normal, it is called "reducing." If a person dislocates their shoulder and their buddy runs up and puts it back in place, it is called "putting it back in place." If you go to the Doctor and THEY put it back in place it is called "reducing." They reduced the dislocated shoulder.

Anyhew, this patient's hernia had actually been there for several years but sometimes this crap just happens to people. The muscles of the abdomen are paper thin and can tear spontaneously with even minimal exertion from being weakened after a traumatic event or even from a medical procedure like being cut through for a surgery. This person had been living with a benign hernia for several years, and for whatever reason it decided to have a shit fit on that particular day. Since the original hernia was nothing new, there was a greater likelihood it could be fixed easily and the doc felt no need for surgical consultation. But the fact it had been recently exacerbated also meant that leaving it be was not the suggested course of action, leading to the aforementioned reduction.

So, to assist the Physician for the reduction I put them in a position called Trendelenburg. In the Trendelenburg position, a patient lies flat and face up with their feet elevated higher than their head. Or the head is dipped below the level of the feet, depending on how you look at it. However, a body remains linear when laying like this. The Merriam-Webster definition says the "pelvis is elevated above the head" with the person's legs hanging over a table . . . semantics. They also claim they are America's most trusted online dictionary for the English language but nobody likes a braggart.

Now what is happening in regard to the hernia fix, is that gravity is assisting in the procedure preparation. The weight of the patient's organs is being pulled away from the hernia and giving the muscles at the hernia site time to relax a bit. I had the patient lay in this position for approximately twenty minutes then let the young Physician know they had been in Trendelenburg for an appropriate amount of time.

The Physician mapped the specifics of the hernia and the offending internal bits then gently massaged the protrusion for several minutes. The patient tolerated the massage and simply laid there while their anatomy was properly realigned. So we're not exactly talking about a day spa massage, it can get uncomfortable. The Physician had moderate success but not total. She used the pneumatic foot lever to raise the bed about a foot higher and then released the air under the upper half of the bed with a different foot lever, in effect increasing the angle of Trendelenburg and returned to massaging.

This had greater success but again, not fully. She still had a department full of patients to manage and multitask, allowing the patient to lay in the new position again. This was for the same reason as the initial, to allow the internal organs to pull away from the hernia and give the muscles surrounding the hernia time to chill out.

She made rounds on her other patients and, true to the circumstances, returned after approximately twenty minutes and resumed the reduction. This time it was a full success. The internal organs had been coerced back to their home. The patient was brought back to a comfortable position of laying flat with their head slightly up this time, instructed to remain comfortable for a while longer. Even though mild, a procedure had been done so the patient needed some monitoring. I occasionally listened to their belly to ensure their internal organs were making appropriate sounds while their job was to report if any new pain developed.

Again, even though it was about as mild as procedures go in the ED, there are still potential adverse effects. A bowel could be twisted or the hernia could tear further. But alas, things went swimmingly from there and the patient was discharged home. Later, I found the Physician and asked about my initial angle to Trendelenburg. I felt as though had I placed the patient in that drastic of an angle initially, the ordeal would have been a single-effort success.

Her answer was the quote mentioned at the start:

"Meh, it's all shades of gray."

A lot of context for what seems like a simple quote, but I had and still have so much appreciation for her words. I would legitimately say that most Physicians are not *that* easy to work with but most are understanding about how the destination from chief complaint to what comes after the ER is rarely ever a simple journey. There are also a few Physicians less willing to have this mindset. There are a few that, if things do not go to their plan, they lose their damn mind. As I have said before, the aspect that I see in nursing that really separates it is how it helps humanize medicine. This not only means that Nurses temporarily wear a teacher hat and bridge the $10 explanation of medicine to a layman's term for people, but it means that Nurses need to wear a psychology hat and figure out the type of Physician they are working with as well.

It is exhausting shit. And that is only the professional aspect. If a Nurse needs something or has to update the provider, they go to the Doctor with gathered evidence. They then use said information to make a suggestion for a proceeding course of action. Here is where the relationship gets pretty dynamic.

If the Physician is personable, they recognize and break down the situation. Sometimes the Nurse's suggestion is spot on, and sometimes there is an angle the Nurse did not consider or realize—It happens. I mean, it's not like the Physician went to a bajillion years of schooling and could see something the Nurse does not. What *is* important is how the Physician handles the situation. Sometimes you work with a super elite Physician and even though the Nurse has a perfectly reasonable suggestion, the Physician will not do it simply because it came from a Nurse. That shit happens. In the scenario where the Nurse doesn't see the whole picture, a good Physician will explain/educate. A rat bastard Physician will belittle and establish that they are the more educated one. Again, it happens. As a Nurse, you need to know what sort of Physician you are working with and learn to approach them in the best interest of the patient. With dickhead docs, I like to present evidence then give them a platform. I will end the scenario with something along the lines of, "What do you think we should do?"

In order to become an emergency room provider (no matter what level): a Medical Doctor, Nurse practitioner, or Physician's assistant, an extensive amount of training in emergency procedures and medicine is required. What is *not* required is passing a stress test. Not a *cardiac* stress test but a test that determines a person's ability to handle when situations go to shit. Because they do; all the time. I have had the displeasure of working with more than one person who turns the department into a hostile work environment that Viking Warlords would have gleaned from with gory approval.

There is a kind of Provider that can whip through the toughest of exams neck and neck with the best of them but then warps into demon mode after the slightest out-of-place patient workup, which holds the key to efficiency in the ER. When providers have this trait, they tend to pinpoint the reason for complications on the RNs. If an EKG doesn't look crystal clear, obviously the RN didn't put leads in the right place, and if the lab results have any abnormality, obviously, the RN doesn't know how to properly draw blood. There are even occasions where a urine sample was not absolutely clean in its collection and a provider places an actual order for urine collection via catheter (time consuming to say the least, which doesn't bode well for all those patients in triage . . . remember them?).

The lack of appeal the situation holds is probably apparent, but still, allow me to enlighten: the procedure involves threading a small tube up a person's urethra (pee hole) to drain the urine. The reason a provider might order this is to ensure there is no bacteria from the person's skin to contaminate the urine sample through the process of naturally urinating. Problem being, the person was an adult in their 30s and completely capable of performing the appropriate hygiene themselves. Just imagine that scenario—walking into a room and looking someone dead in the eye and saying you need to thread a tube up their urethra because the Doctor said so. Pressing the provider's request would get a Nurse smacked and it might be the only time I would stand back and think of how well deserved it was.

These providers have a demonic presence hidden in plain sight, even under the best of circumstances. Now think of what the ER is. It is an entire department designed to welcome the collective of society when they malfunction. From its foundation, it is a place that operates off the understanding that things are not going to go right, that most days simply managing the chaos is the best way through.

Life, limb, or eyesight.

Take three steps back with me to triage, and I will explain a situation that highlights "malfunction" in its purest form—a situation where a patient's fingers got jammed and a situation that is otherwise a couple days of ice packs and over-the-counter ibuprofen that turned into finger strangulation to the point of potential lossage. The X-Factors from "Ouch!" to

"Amputation" were the thick skull and dragon rings he was wearing. The triage RN immediately recognized the situation and got his hand in an ice water bath and labeled his electronic chart appropriately: "Needs to see the provider *immediately*." He was one of those jerks that had a 30-second triage wait, breezing past the chief complaints of muscle strains and constipation.

The chaos of the events overshadow what exactly happened to his fingers in my memory so the mechanism of injury, I do not recall. What stood out was how his rings complicated the swelling process that naturally occurs with injury. They needed to be removed and by the look of them, it is questionable if he would have been able to naturally remove them on any given day so they needed to be cut off. He wasn't 100% sure of their material but thought they were tungsten; either way, the ring cutting tool in the department didn't stand a chance. The RN and the tech set up a system to tag each other out of cutting away at the rings because of how time consuming it was. Each ring would grind down three cutting tools before making their way through a single one of them . . . and he had four.

The tension of the situation was compounded when the patient experienced increasing pain, not only from the inflamed fingers but also the extra pressure and movement of the ring cutters. We did our due diligence and made sure that there were no broken bones before getting to work. The patient was begging and pleading for the staff to discontinue their efforts because of how bad it hurt. The provider was kept informed of the situation and extremely reluctant to order anything more than ibuprofen for the pain—eventually giving in when the patient and family in the room exploded in anger at the lack of attention to pain combined with the relentless efforts to remove the rings.

When the department realized they did not have enough cutting tools to get through all the rings, they placed an SOS call out to local EMS as well as their sister hospitals. EMS crews showed up with the cutting tools from their rigs, all of which either failed faster than the ER's or simply could not fit around the bulk of the rings. A hospital in the same network had a specialized electronic cutting tool that was used in their surgical department and paged for a medical courier to deliver the instrument with an ETA of 60 minutes.

The patient was down to his last ring by that point, and despite witnessing the immediate return of circulation and subsequent pain relief, refused to push forward. The department was out of tools and waiting for the electronic tool which was still approximately 45 minutes out. He could no longer take it . . . he was tapping out.

Yes, people don't understand what help looks like, and yes, people don't understand there is rarely a pain free option—some people don't understand that getting better isn't a pretty process. They "know" what is right in front of them. What was right in front of this patient was not two fingers with relief, it was one finger pushed past its threshold for pain. Both the patient and the father were steadfast in that they did not want to keep going because they "did not think it would be like this."

Also worth noting: it is absolutely illegal to touch a patient if they are refusing treatment while of sound mind—all arguments to debate the faculties of a person refusing to continue (when a finger is at stake) would be given an audience in my humble opinion, however, he only had his father bending his ear. Medically speaking, he was not under the influence or suffering brain damage so he could indeed "reasonably" make decisions.

The patient and family signed an AMA (Against Medical Advice). In short, that's a patient's way of saying "This is not how I thought it would be." And, after signing, they're free to go because of free will. If you think that happens easily, you're wrong. The tech, the RN, and the Charge RN all expressed heavy grievance that day at the idea of leaving with the last ring intact. Delay tactics to educate the patient and his family failed with about 15 minutes left for the other tool to arrive.

In this particular situation, in the eyes of the provider, the escalating situation and loss of control was the fault of one RN. *Can you guess who?* The under-matched equipment, the patient/family lack of patience, the crumbling tolerance to pain (with minimal management) of the methods needed to fix the situation . . . was the RN's fault. The RN had not acted fast enough and the "window was lost" to appropriately combat the inflammation. The RN should have done more to educate the patient and their family to ensure compliance. Yet wouldn't you know it? I lived to work another day—learning from the good, the bad, the ugly, and the skull and crossbones rings of finger death.

And while the ring incident was urgent, pushing emergent, the point is that Physicians are the lead in the department, the amount of truly emergent situations that go according to plan without any sort of pivoting, setback, or failure are nearly nonexistent. There is enough guilt to go around after efforts fail trying to infuse blood into a person fast enough to keep pace with what is being lost. Or when someone's heart picks your shift to finally give out for good. When a patient comes barreling through the bay doors with the ambulance lights still blinding waves of blue flashes behind them on their way in, one of those moments where all the additional training and knowledge comes clicking together for a Nurse, a Doctor, EMT and despite everything done right and in haste the person dies. It might be one of a small number of things those drama shows get right that the team still has to rally and know that there are dozens of other people that need their attention.

Situations like these are when Nurses feel like they are being drawn and quartered. When patients and family members come apart at the seams, that is enough by itself . . . but to have your coworkers (who you're just trying to support in the same fight) deliver scathing remarks on your performance . . . it just seems unnecessary. But again, that's where the "malfunctioning humans" part comes back into focus. We are all malfunctioning and we are all capable of losing our cool. So, from situation to situation, will you push forward with resilience, doing what is right and to the best of your ability, even when ridicule is a possibility at the end of it all? As with the point of view from the ER bed, you never know if there are three or four other rooms currently building a Nurse's resilience

As much as I disagree with the Provider who can't handle a less-than-perfect scenario, at least most of them show up each day to see their patients . . . I want to give credit where credit is due. Facing the fiery attitude of patients is a hit or miss ordeal for those who call the shots. I used to absolutely *hate* getting yelled at by patients. Not because I can't take a verbal, but because it bothered me that I was breaking my back trying to help and the response I got was ugliness. What compounds this frustration is that most people understand there is a type of hierarchy in the ER—in any medical setting. They know that there are only a few Doctors (hell, at some ERs only one) so they simply cannot be in the trenches like the Nurses. It doesn't work. Nurses are the workhorses, but people don't understand the extent of it. Without Nurses, the place would cave in. There is ALWAYS some form of the statement, "You are in here all the time, I have only seen the Doctor once" that lets me know I have been putting in great effort to provide care.

It may seem like a moot point, but there are some who don't realize Nurses didn't go to medical school. Therefore, Nurses don't have the right initials behind their name to order a lot of things and they don't dictate the overall direction of care yet Nurses are an integral part of that and through assessments and communication, and provide valuable information on how/where the direction is steered. Alas, at the end of the day, it is the Physician that plots the destination.

Trust me, Nurses have caught way too many fists throughout their careers and if they had the final say on plotting the path forward, the issue would be addressed immediately. Anytime a patient came in with a trio of police because they decided violence was the best option out of a situation that person would have a trio of sedating medications in circulation to replace the police from the initial, "fuck you" thrown out to the staff.

And that is under the better circumstances. Enter a scenario where a patient is aggressive, assaulting, or even just belligerent—sometimes it comes short of an act of God to get a Nurse backup.

I am not saying that all Providers hide from tense situations, I am just saying there seems to be a negative correlation between the level of aggression from a patient and the face-to-face time between them and the doc. There is an internal back and forth I go through when it comes to violent patients. The medical aspect of me completely understands we cannot exactly give out sedative shots to people at every sign of anger in the department. It is utterly inappropriate medicine to toss a knockout shot into any patient for a quickly managed issue whenever they throw a fit, besides, we would run out of the meds for when we really need them.

All I am saying is that from a human standpoint, I *am* tired of excess aggression and violence. It is unbelievable. I wish I used that word, "unbelievable" in a manner of "Wow, that is amazing" but I don't. I really don't. I mean it in a manner of the exhausted "Are you fucking kidding me?" exhaled into hands covering my face. Years ago, I would have never guessed that a fully grown adult would check into the Emergency Room because of such bad gout pain they could not drive to the pharmacy to pick up their prescription, but be able to drive to the ER. On top of that, think the best way to get the immediate pain relief they desired was to berate the Nurse for everything they did that was not actively handing them pain medications (vital signs, assessment, chart, etc).

Situations like that are an easy "in and out" scenario so yeah, the answer is definitely not to do something that would keep that sort of awful in the department a minute longer than necessary. What sucks is that, in a busy ER, something like that is likely not going to be seen anytime soon. So, the RN is stuck face-to-face with the occasional raging bull for a few hours. Sometimes, the situation is where the storm is brewing and the patient escalates their aggression and doubles down on their situation which necessitates a long stay in the ER. Perhaps they have a condition that requires reevaluation at least once before a decision is going to be made, or even more so, a very common occurrence is where the it is known that the patient will be staying in the hospital, however, there are no beds at the inn so the ER becomes their hospital stay (read on). This patient will be in the ER for hours, I mean HOURS, like so many hours that it turns into days, meanwhile the Physicians' station to do their work will be literally across the hall from a patient spewing their displeasure of the situation so loud that the floor above them can hear it and the Doctor will not address the situation until the explosion event.

Even here, what typically happens is the patient gets a child's dose of meds to calm them or manage their pain. Again, the fear being, if they get too much of a med, they won't be able to leave the ER because they will be too doped up or even potentially go so far as to need assistance breathing. It is one of those deals where if you give a medication to 10 different people with every aspect about the medication the same such as dose, route, etc, each of the 10 people will have different degrees of efficacy. So, there is a chance that a medication designed to relax a person could be given to a person so sensitive to it that they need assistance breathing. It is a nightmare contradiction that occurs multiple times every day in every ER. In an ER Nurses's order of operations, the ideal sunset ending is . . . well, a patient scooting off to wherever they end up just so long as no punches get thrown.

Okay, well, I say that but just like if you travel around the country, world, wherever, being in an ER you will meet the same handful of nursing personalities. One of them is indeed the jackass who is all about a tussle. The hardass that has no problem with rowdy patients and does no form of de-escalation, they know that they will have backup if an alert is called. These Nurses are a-holes and unfortunately they are out there. These Nurses are trouble as is but doubled down when a patient will come in for the sole purpose of wanting a bed to sleep in and food in their belly. When these patients come in and it is time to send them on their way, they will oftentimes attempt the "well you didn't investigate my 15 other complaints" route and when that fails because they are told to go see a family Doctor for their joint pain, they turn to violence. "I am in an Emergency room, right!? Are you telling me you don't help people here!?" Most Nurses will bob and weave the verbal assault that follows but the aggressive Nurse will head straight in George Foreman style metaphorically and eventually literally.

In any other situation, this type of Nurse is one of those "strong personality" Nurses that is really just an unlikable asshole. The ones that social media praises as the "angry Nurse but will save your ass in an emergency." The reality here is that these Nurses are dangerous. They are dangerous because they are never wrong and if there is any place you want to work with a sense of humility, it is in the ER. These Nurses are also typically younger and usually not only the ones that are constantly bringing up how they are only going to be in the ER for a couple years while they go to Nurse Anesthetist school. As you have likely surmised, they are also typically the ones who avoid signing up for patients that involve a lot of nitty gritty work, "riff raff" patients to them. They jump on the trauma patients, the cardiac arrest patients. Basically, patients that will have a swarm of other disciplines involved and are typically in and out of the ER within an hour.

If this type of patient is given to the "avoids confrontation Nurse", they still have their discharge delayed by an hour at least because the Nurse is too afraid to object to their verbal assault and will instead make repeated trips back to the Doctor updating them on the patient's complaints until eventually the flat out notice that the patient does not have an emergent complaint and thus will not be having any further testing or examination done. By this point the Charge Nurse is typically hounding the patient's Nurse as to why the patient is still occupying a room and pressuring the Nurse to discharge the patient. It is a pretty regular occurrence, there are a handful of ways the situation can play out, anywhere from the Nurse bribing patient out with a bag full of sandwiches, snacks, and cans of pop (if the department even has any) to the patient packing up and leaving but definitely making sure the entire department, Nurses, Doctors, patients, and families all are well informed of their displeasure and having security in tow.

Usually, this type of Nurse isn't terrible to work with but they can bog down the ER by not having figured out a decent work/empathy balance. I can appreciate that they treat their patients like human beings but also when they actually listen to the entirety of every patient's chief complaint monologue, they leave their coworkers drowning.

Most Nurses have dealt with the unsatisfied customer situation regularly enough even within their first month on the job that they no longer have the patience for shenanigans and will come prepared. They will run through the entire workup that was completed in the ER, make sure the patient knows that any lingering complaint is to be taken to their primary Doctor, and that the ER stay is in fact complete. When the rebuttal comes up, the Discharge Instruction to take non-emergency complaints to a family Doctor is reiterated. Done. End of it. There are equal chances that the patient will leave in any form of mood but also equally that they will roll over and go back to sleep. This is where the nursing is over and unfortunately, a security escort is brought in. The completely asinine thing is that if a patient TRULY does not want to leave the ER, which is a very regular occurrence, the police will get called in to arrest the patient for trespassing. If it seems ridiculous, it is because it is. But what is even more ridiculous is that if the patient complains of literally anything medical at all, the police will not be allowed to take the patient without a Physician's note saying that the patient was examined and has no medical need to be in the Emergency Room. Triple down on the ridiculousness if the patient strikes up a mental health complaint. More on that later.

Just like the previous paragraph begins, this is most Nurses. They have figured out how to move with speed and efficiency. Not much to say about them, they just want to work and go the fuck home. They take the wins and manage the losses.

CHANGING SHIFT

Talk to any Nurse, doesn't even have to be ER & they will swear there is a dark magic that surrounds any type of transitioning period. If a patient is going to start decompensating from their illness or injury, it will happen as the shift comes to a close or right after a note on a patient's response to anything performed. It is the damndest thing. If you are a Nurse and you are reading this, your immediate thought is the "it happened in the elevator" scenario. That is (usually) no lie. Patients will wait until the least opportune moment to have anything happen all the way from pissing themselves or throat reclosing from that allergic reaction that had been well managed for four hours - legit, those examples made the cut because they have happened to me.

Whether it is giving the doc an update or a report on a current patient's status to prepare them for transport up to their new room. Upon completion, they will have a respiratory rate that is 15 breaths per minute faster, their oxygen will be tanking, their blood pressure might as well read "garbage over dead" and they will have rolled over three times in bed twisted in their IV tubing with the IV ripped out and covered in piss or shit. Always covered in piss or shit, seriously.

When Nurses give their patient over to another Nurse, whether it be for the change of shift to the next unfortunate soul in the ER or sending a patient to their post ER destination, we give a rundown of main topics called a patient report. Reiterating that the ER is a continual motion machine, we focus on what emergency situation has brought the patient to the hospital, their current state of being, and the important events that have taken place since then. So essentially: how they were, how they are now, and highlights of how they got from A to B. We aren't regurgitating the memoir the patient used as their story in triage.

Emergency Nurses don't give a shit about the last time our patients took a shit. Only unless they are checked into the ER for a problem with shitting, which actually, yeah, it does happen a lot more than you would think, it is trivial. On that note, it may surprise or depress you on just how many times people-like full grown adult people in their 30s-check into the ER because they haven't pooped in a day. People mess with it, too. Please, stop touching your poop, people. Just stop. I feel like I shouldn't have to say that but in nursing it happens a lot. We call them "Poopcasso" patients. They don't poop at home so they come to the ER, get some meds and for reasons unbeknownst to anyone, would rather poop in the ER-or more accurately, the ER bed-then scoop it up and present it to the Nurse.

Anyway, unlike the above paragraph, quick and to the point is what the call to the next Nurse should be. It isn't that things like a patient's bowel habits and skin issues aren't important. They are. It is as simple as how I mentioned that the ER serves a different purpose. Our job is to get the ball rolling on correcting that blood glucose of 700, the metabolic derangement, the seizure, allergic reaction, etc.

Unfortunately, what the Nurse *then* needs to include about the patient is a blurb on their temperament. How that has become necessary information says *something* about our society, not sure exactly what exactly, but definitely something. For nursing purposes, it is a safety item. Handing off a patient to the next Nurse now involves discussing things like how much blood a person has lost and been replaced, what sort of neurological functioning a person has, what sort of rhythm their heart is in, how many medications are required to maintain their blood pressure, and how much oxygen they are requiring to stay alive—oh, and the fact that they cussed out the Nurse for bringing them nitro for their chest pain instead of Dilaudid.

If there is one area I wish I could speak freely to patients it is about the uncomfortable means of recovery. I told you, there is rarely a pain free option, but some people take it to the extreme and threaten physical harm to the staff for things like running a swab in their nose to check for the flu when the patient comes in with flu-like symptoms. These people should have a conversation with patients that need a special means of hemorrhage management called a Rhino Rocket; it is basically shoving tampons up your nose to stop a severe nosebleed. Or if they had to be restrained because the neck brace was uncomfortable and they put the spinal cord territory in their neck at too great of a risk when they ripped off the brace. People don't give two shits about the femur sticking up through their quadriceps muscles, the meth and alcohol in their system did as much as any pain killer we could give them. Oh, but that neck brace! That thing is always too much to handle. I wish these drama class dropout patients could have an open discussion with family members that were in that same room two hours before them and talk about what the silence was like after someone they had known and loved for decades died in the very bed they currently occupy. Maybe compare notes on the pain they are going through.

I have tried to lace this entire book with various forms of humor but one area I *do* take seriously is that we need a generational change on how we view death. I wish we could start learning, from a young age, to have a better emotional relationship with death—not to be confused with mourning the loss of loved ones—but simply not to wait until that loss occurs to begin the road to peace and to spend more of our emotions and energy celebrating that we got to have certain people in our lives instead of fear, grief, disbelief—basically the path to the dark side. I say this in regards to working in emergency medicine . . . when a person becomes chronically ill or experiences a worsening of their chronic condition (called acute or chronic). So many times people that have lived long enough with years of strain on their vital organs, they will have what is called a DNR/DNI, which means Do Not Resuscitate/Do Not Intubate.

It means do not put that person through the trauma of keeping them alive. The trauma of multiple pokes from drawing blood and establishing IVs, broken ribs and breastbone from CPR to keep their blood pumping. It means do not put a tube in their throat and have a machine breath for them. It means when something life threatening happens, allow the natural process to take place. It means the person has had a heartfelt discussion with loved ones and Physicians and they have come to the decision that should anything happen to them either the efforts to save them would be too drawn out and they don't want to spend their remaining days looking like a shadow government alien autopsy project or their quality of life after the incident would not be expected to return to anything they would value.

The dicey territory comes when a family member is placed in charge of making decisions for a patient; when this time comes, they are unable to honor the DNR/DNI wishes. It is not my place to say this is right or wrong. That is not what is happening here. What I am saying is that from the inside of those walls, we all feel better about the situation when we aren't filling the room with the sounds of alarms blaring because they don't detect signs of life. Nobody wants to witness the crunch and crack of ribs breaking through efforts to reel in that thousand yard stare look on someone's face while another team of people crank back their head and put that tube down their throat. Nobody feels good about creating burn marks on a person by sending two hundred joules of electricity through someone's chest cavity every other minute, especially knowing that the likelihood of success is nil. Does "dying with dignity" mean dying with more tubes putting their waste products on display by pulling the last thing a person ate out of their stomach and into canisters? Loss of bowel control? Having a urine bag hanging on the bed railing down by their dusky feet?

The right answer is unique to each and every person, every family. The troublesome topic is that when a DNR/DNI is in place, the plan to make that official is not done with a faint heart. And while our job is the medical aspect of saving lives and improving health, there are no hard lines separating how a person feels about things and it is not our place to say what is right and what is wrong in the heat of that moment but we honestly cannot help but wonder if it was worth it.

That is the final word on Putting a Plan together. There are pragmatic elements throughout—from Gathering Info to Communication Standards—but again, in the end, the goal is an efficient patient experience. It is important to keep in mind that the ER isn't a day out with your best friends. An efficient experience isn't always going to garnish a 5 star Yelp review. That's pretty much the endgame of this book, remember? But sometimes the patient is yourself—is *ourselves*—and we need to be willing to operate on ourselves in order to grow as a human. There is a jackass inside all of us, but don't just let it sit there. Kick the damn mule and get it going in the desired direction. Put a Plan Together and make your way toward a desired destination.

PART 5: PROBLEM BEHIND THE PAIN

If nursing was transparent enough about the politics involved in the medical industry, there would likely be an increase in attrition rate just from learning about that shit. So to kick off the "problem behind the pain" let's look at another "P" word, and you might've guessed it: Politics.

A special type of nightmare is when the hospital is full. No rooms at the Inn. Patients will simply stay in the ER room until something opens up. This beautiful clusterfuck makes taking care of patients a royal pain in the ass because they are technically but not physically moving on in their hospital stay which means the focus of their care shifts from emergency to maintenance. ER Nurses are not experienced in maintenance (i.e. fix, stabilize, move on). From a high level standpoint, the patients are still in the ER, except they are under a different Doctor's care. If a patient is in this situation and has a need that is not addressed with the current orders, the Nurse then consults a matrix of which Doctor is working. There are admitting Doctors who will solely do the admission process for generic patients, then the hospitalist, the intensivist for critically ill patients, then Doctors for any specialty like cardiac, pulmonary, surgical, etc.

If there is any sort of weird voodoo that holds consistency for these situations, it is that issues like a "full hospital house" typically exist around *larger* scale issues that affect the entire geographical region-weather is usually a good enough example. A blizzard increases emergency accidents and exacerbates people's chronic conditions causing them to herd to the ER like The Walking Dead zombies saunter towards anything with a pulse. The ER team gets caught in this shift that becomes twelve hours of tug-of-war between the patients using the ER as their hospital room for the night and the fresh onslaught of chief complaints funneling into the department. Nursing becomes this dichotomy of "ER Nursing" such as assisting the Physician with a quick sedation procedure to retrieve a chunk of steak that got caught in a person's throat and "Med Pass" such as assisting patients with their appropriate medication. I honestly don't know how people have room for breakfast or dinner with the pharmacy sized amount of medications they take.

Lord help the Nurse should they need anything at all before the admission orders are placed. And double down on the help if the admission takes place within an hour either direction of the Doctors' change of shift. Cue the elevator waiting music. Of course, the ER Doctor that is physically present at the time will usually assist if it is an emergency. The Nurse rarely escapes the Physician's . . . let's call it a 'request' to "Contact the right Doctor." It is a lame circumstance where there's a gap in the patient's handoff and needs to change because given the right temperament from the Physician and the wrong confidence from the Nurse, an emergent situation might not get the proper attention.

And as for that matrix? Just trying to figure out *which* Doctor to get a hold of—a mind numbing process that should be anything but. A multitude of Doctors can be assigned to take on a patient's case. Nurses will check to see who is the overnight doc, message them, and get a response that they are *not* in fact the person to consult, they are Dr. X and the Nurse needs to get in touch with Doctor Y. Doctor Y will then message back saying the Nurse needs to check with Dr. Z for this particular concern. The Nurse will *then* message the Dr. Z who *then* typically tells the Nurse not to reach out to them over such inappropriate things. If a Nurse is lucky, they will basically be told to reach out to Dr. Z's student. The entire charade takes place over roughly two hours of messaging back and forth while the patient is crafting numerous comment cards on how awful the place is because they are stuck in the tiny hospital bed and haven't gotten their nightly wind down medication cocktail. All the best nursing care in the country flies out the window because of . . . well, politics.

Specialty Doctors are hit or miss. They either love coming to consult in the ER or they loathe it. They show up and greatly assist the patient, typically teaching the ER staff a thing or two along the way. Or they show up many hours later (had to finish that dinner reservation) and toss work environment grenades up and down the joint. They are used to working out of their office and have a staff they are used to working with, which creates for their own well-oiled machine. The ER is the streets of Baghdad in their eyes and even though the Nurses are there to help, they don't know the ins-and-outs of how the specialist likes things done. In addition, they have five or six other patients they need to attend to, so the specialist has their rhythm thrown off even more when they don't have a team of Nurses to manage some of the things they don't typically have to. On these nights (so basically in the ER), it's the Nurse's ass whenever literally anything goes wrong. Or at least there are plenty of parties out there who will try to make it seem that way.

Many Physicians have no problem expressing their displeasure with the nursing staff, too. Eating and drinking is undoubtedly the most common "nursing infraction." Even though the patient was repeatedly educated they were not to eat or drink anything until the results were in on their workup, or to refrain from eating and drinking until the Physician had arrived and completed a procedure, they ate an entire sub sandwich complete with chips and a large drink their family brought them. It doesn't matter that the RN was managing a dozen other things at once, all that matters is that the Nurse did not teleport across the ER and physically smack that Jimmy Johns BLT out of the patient's hands.

If the patient doesn't have family to break the rules for them, the Nurse is in for a long shift of begging. At its worst, the patient might whine, complain, or cry that water is a necessity for life and then try to declare how shit of a Nurse they have because they obviously don't understand basic concepts like dehydration. I wish I were joking about such an occasion. I *wish* that kind of scenario was made up.

Nursing and the politics included is just like any other industry: do more (and more efficiently) with less. It doesn't matter that the industry is people and that people have nil consistency about them. I mean, have you ever taken a Sociology class? It's barely a science, a 40% consistency with a social experiment is considered a win. That's failing by a large margin elsewhere. The strain on Nurses at bedside is obvious —we are spread thin. Nurses are the ones getting our hands dirty, wearing smartwatches chiming with the ten thousandth step *way* too early into a shift, managing complex medical illnesses that affect complex medical histories. And juggling detail-oriented tasks and not getting distracted with every call that rings asking for an accommodation for the ER to be more like things the patient has at home. Still, if anything goes wrong, it easily falls on the ER Nurse.

Charting by itself is tedious but necessary, the saying goes "if you didn't chart it then it didn't happen." Charting needs to tell the tale of what happened during a patient's stay in the ER. However, charting is getting to the point where it is nearly equal to the amount of time a Nurse spends actually taking care of their patient. Plus, more and more of a Nurse's time is spent charting deviations and exceptions to the plan. The ER by nature is a collection of imperfect situations, the opposite of perfect, really, and with any imperfection that happens, it has to be explained no matter the cause. Explaining things like, how their patient who checked in with pneumonia has a "low oxygen reading because they don't like wearing the oxygen tubing and frequently remove it." Or "The patient wants to get up and walk to use the restroom because they have been in the ER bed for hours", even though they are in the ER for exacerbated heart failure and pass out after minimal activity. The clash of being acutely sick with wanting things to be familiar puts patient safety in ever present crosshairs. If that shot ever lines up, even if ever so briefly, management will get involved in some way.

It is a bit shameful to admit but also utterly honest, that there are times when Nurses will worry about if a lifesaving measure was charted properly on the same level as if it were performed properly. The repercussions of charting can range from understandable, to annoying, to severe. Under the best of scenarios, management will email the Nurse about the situation days later to ask if the Nurse explicitly educated the patient or reinforced the education by writing the instructions on the white board every room contains. They will run through a checklist of error safety net actions and ask for the Nurse's side of the story.

Under less ideal circumstances, they will actually walk through the department at change of shift and wander around to "rub elbows" and make small talk with the ones in the trenches when their real purpose is to locate a particular Nurse in a manner that is all too reminiscent of that wandering family member by lazily catching eyes with their target RN and using that as the tractor beam to close in and initiate the conversation about the real purpose for being there-to mention those labs that were drawn late or whatever.

Ultimately, management is there for patient safety, sure, but for whatever reason *ahem—money* the answer is rarely to implement strategies that make the overall working environment actually safer. The answer is to implement new management strategies and checklists, or hang up reminder flyers or add a new notification armband to place on your patient. Things get so congested and nothing feels particularly important when everything is supposed to be the most important thing.

FLAVOR OF THE MONTH

Every couple of years, there is a new gig that sweeps corporate America as the next "it" thing in the medical field. At one point in time, it was these fucking white boards. I honestly hate that I hate them because as mentioned above, they are indeed a great tool. I truly believe that knowledge is power and in a critical scenario, going over the plan with your patient, and using the white board as a visual, is real time multimedia. They *do* help patients, however, they quickly became a management fad. The white boards have some acronym on them like HEART or whatever the choice of that hospital is. AIDIT is the one that was the most ridiculous, when we were meeting out patients they wanted us to "A"cknowledge the patient, "I"ntroduce ourselves and give a heads up of other staff that might enter the room (there were little pictures of colored scrub tops on the white board with references to which department like XRay wears which color), "D"iscuss the plan . . . cannot remember the second I, but the T was to "T"hank the patient . . . for what? Couldn't tell you.

Doing things like investigating faulty whiteboard protocol is the shit people who haven't worn scrubs to the hospital in seven or more years have hype dreams over—it's their Superbowl corridor scenario, like "THIS IS WHAT WE PLAY FOR!" It doesn't matter the shift a Nurse is having either. They could have a person with blood in all the wrong parts of their body as well as on the floor get saved from the grips of death and taken up to the ICU. The manager would debrief you on the situation with a quick "nice job" on saving the person's life but then have a 5-minute lecture on how you could have updated the white board in a more proficient manner.

Another one is when patients are discharged home, they receive Home Care Instructions. Discharge Instructions are what they have been called since long before I had the horrible thought in my head of, "Yeah, maybe I'll go to Nursing School and make a difference." However, a couple years ago that corporate America good idea bus took an unfortunate turn through the hospital I was working at and decided to call the Discharge Instructions an "After Visit Summary." Heaven and Earth help you if you called them Discharge Instructions to your patient and management was eavesdropping on your time going over the paperwork.

Both scenarios—the white board and the Discharge Instructions—are potential pitfalls that will get you pulled aside by someone in management for an education on why those two items are necessary. Meanwhile, you have 4-5 other patients with mounting needs. Ask any Nurse you know and there are Vegas odds you will be in disbelief. And I mean disbelief like the Merriam-Webster type of disbelief.

Imagine a situation where you have been running tirelessly for 12 hours, bouncing between five forms of the same, "why is it so cold in here?", "do you know how long I've been waiting?", and "that pain medication doesn't work on me, I told the Doctor I wanted a different one" statements with only one small breather of a break and maybe a few extra minutes squeezed in to go to the restroom yourself. You do this for forty hours within three days. Then the next time you come into the same place to do it all over again, you have an email from someone who hasn't worn scrubs to work for probably 15 years, reprimanding you because one of the patients you had to give blood to had improper documentation. The vital signs are supposed to be taken every fifteen minutes and you chart one of the sets of vital signs at fourteen minutes.

It happens weekly. And yes, that example made the writing because it happened to me. I charged vital signs at a 14-minute mark after a blood transfusion had ended, which, per protocol, is supposed to be 15 minutes. If a Nurse is lucky, that is the end of it, read an email, sign a statement acknowledging the "education" and move on. If a Nurse is unlucky, they will have to do some remedial training. When? It is usually at the least convenient time possible.

To reiterate, patient safety is a must, truly is. But the CYA (Cover Your Ass) in Nursing has nearly gotten to the point of disrupting care. Additional example: if a person has a blood clot, they get an infusion initiated that is designed to break apart the clot. As a result, a natural side effect of this is the potential to bleed. There are markers in the blood that are routinely tested to ensure that the medication level is not getting dangerously high. If that happens, then the patient is at a tremendous risk for either spontaneously bleeding uncontrollably or having an uncontrollable bleed from what would otherwise be a normal bleed—for instance, if a person trips and falls, they get a bruise. If a person with *this* kind of medication trips and falls? They get a hematoma: a collection of blood because those banged up blood vessels just won't quit bleeding. It is a simple comparison but can be dangerous if that collection of blood is in your brain. Bad day.

The risk of the necessity is mitigated by checking the blood for its clotting properties every couple of hours. Now, a slight abnormality of a little longer time to clot is okay, and it is expected because we are doing it. But a problem I have run into is that the lab results will get flagged as "elevated" because they are using a normal person as the scale. However, not only does the lab ask if the person has a medication that would alter the results, there is even a protocol one would follow to adjust the medication based on altered results. Now, with outstanding results, part of the hospital protocol is that the Doctor needs to be notified, which is a safety measure. Common things are severely elevated like blood sugar, cardiac markers, electrolytes, etc.

Extremely abnormal results could indicate life or death and the Physician would need to be notified.

Now, in this instance, the elevated result was expected, so the charting reflected that the Provider was not notified and the protocol was followed. From the Nursing Management's point of view, the Provider was still supposed to be notified because they did not specifically write an order to not notify them of the expected abnormal results. Yes, that is indeed as ridiculous as it initially reads. You may need to read it another time or two and it will still be equally true and ridiculous. Systems are getting to the point of flagging these results or even recorded vital signs, so they will make you acknowledge and chart actions taken on potential issues like those damn pop-ups or widgets that assault you when all you're trying to do is go online and look up movie showtimes.

For example, take sepsis as an occurrence. Sepsis is an infection that could have begun anywhere but now has run rampant throughout a person's body—doesn't have to be a surgical or blood infection per se, like all those midnight settlement commercials bait people into believing. There are warning signs for this all the way from microscopic events that are revealed through labs or obviously observable things like an elevated temperature, heart rate, or even confusion . . . very generic things that could paint the picture of a septic patient. Some of these findings could also fit the narrative of a person who just jogged a couple miles to start their day. The system doesn't know the difference, but it still tries to identify trends of serious ailments and alerts the staff with pop-ups that don't allow any charting until the warning pop-up is acknowledged and some sort of commentary made about what is going to be done about it, like the person is not in the hospital. And sometimes with sick patients, their irregular findings persist for days to weeks.

Yet there aren't flags and warnings for things like when a patient has concerning trends shown on serial EKGs. Where the answer is buried for reasons like that, who knows. There was a huge campaign called Surviving Sepsis initiated in 2002 (I believe) so it could be that it is just the "it" topic throughout the upper echelon levels of healthcare—not to downplay sepsis, it *is* sneaky and serious. Prevention is the best care so while the little alerts are annoying, their purpose is understood. The confusion comes from why *that* versus other things and also how much of a pain in the ass it makes charting at times.

Electronic scanning is something Nurses have a love/hate relationship with. It really has become a dominant feature in patient safety. However, when Nurses are on the move, especially in emergent scenarios, it can be a challenge. Patients wear wristbands printed when they check in, the wristband is unique to their stay and contains personal information such as: name, date of birth and a generated number unique to their current visit. It also has a barcode on it which certainly does not help the Nurse when the patient is paranoid that Nurses are doing things just to rack up the bill.

Again, it is born out of patient safety but has its flaws and is another miniature battle that can be one of the thousand cuts in a Nurse's shift that can drag a good shift to a shit shift. The idea is to serve as an additional safety check to verify that they are the right patient for the med, procedure, whatever. These wristbands need to be scanned in order to digitally "grant access" (so to speak) to administering medications. Sometimes they are faded and don't read, sometimes the whole damn scanner doesn't work and the Nurse dives into one of those roles they never thought they would become: a damn electronics repairman, who, let's be honest here, turns it off and back on usually does it but still it takes time.

Confused, elderly, withdrawing patients, become a wacky waving inflatable arm flailing tube man. It's like trying to lasso a calf at the rodeo just to do your first of multiple patient-safety checks or a horribly misplaced carnival game. But 99 times out of 100, scanning is a great thing. It's those times when it is not working for some reason, especially in a truly emergent scenario. The second aspect of scanning after the patient is the medication to make sure it is correct based on what the Doctor ordered. And in very modern hospitals, if a medication pump is used, the pump itself has a barcode that is integrated into the system. If anything between these three items doesn't jive, then it is a massive hiccup, it can delay life saving treatment. Yet 80% of the time, when a Nurse is clocking 10,000 steps managing an ER overcrowded with mundane complaints, it is another delay. An acceptable price for patient safety, but still another reason that adds seconds between a Nurse coming back around to check on a different patient.

In emergency scenarios, Nurses do what needs to be done: give a med emergently to save someone and enter the medication into the pump manually? Great, it needs to be done when it needs to be done, someone's life was on the line. But when the storm clears, if there are med discrepancies, it's time again for CYA. So to make sure everything that was given is accounted for and documented appropriately, you have to retrace your steps which will take five times as long as it should. The road to Hell is paved with good intentions, as they say.

Starting to get a decent idea of the problem behind the pain? The aforementioned pages provide a conglomerate of anecdotes (some personal) and unfortunate realities that lie behind the facade of a typical ER experience or set of ER presuppositions. Now . . . the pages that *follow* will zoom out in scope onto a nationwide buzzsaw that was the beginning of COVID-19, in the Year of Our Lord 2020. And Lord . . . what a year it was.

Instead of reliving that time (because who in the hell would want to do that?), let's examine the problem it all exposed behind the pain of an ailing medical industry.

COVID-19

I would be remiss if I didn't address the nature of patient care in a post-2020 (read: COVID-19) . As fate would have it, I actually transitioned into the ICU in November of 2019. This transition was accompanied by pretty decent training, and was actually much more what I was hoping nursing school would have been like. Training at this specific hospital was applicable and integrated with actual working shifts alongside someone to orient oneself into the department. It would have been nearly perfect had it not been for the "classroom" portion—the part closest to goddamn nursing school. It is unreal how nursing academics just cannot get it figured out.

During class (which was just once a week for three months, along with regularly scheduled shifts & online modules) we'd go over that week's online module which usually wound up as 50% "Let me tell you how cool I am" and 50% arts & crafts time . . . like kindergarten. Yes, some of our grade was based on creativity behind making poster boards, skits, videos, etc. and as a person in my early 30s, it all felt pretty unbearable. I assumed everyone else would have thought the same, but I was horribly off base. The other Nurses I was with fucking loved this kind of bullshit. But hey . . . to each his or her own

Anyway, the point of this section is to acknowledge the environment leading up to COVID and its aftermath. I remember one specific evening in early 2020. It was in our pre-shift huddle, and some of us Nurses were talking about an internet meme we saw of a guy kneeling down, chugging a Corona beer and the caption read something along the lines of "If This Is How I Get Coronavirus, Sign Me Up." We all looked at each other and admitted that we had no clue what Coronavirus was, so we looked online and there was maybe one news article from a generic news app that hardly mentioned Coronavirus so we all shrugged and went about our day. That was early February 2020. Little did we know, by the end of that same month, the hallways in the ICU would look like a broadway musical wardrobe. There were supply carts and isolation gear such as gowns, masks, and ventilation hoods hanging tripled up on hooks outside rooms. Typically, these things are single use and disposable. Everyone knows from the news that hospitals were overwhelmed. But little things that don't typically make the headlines are details like how Nurses were using disposable protective equipment not only as shared amongst other Nurses, but for weeks on end. Single-use Personal Protective Equipment quickly became abused like a hockey player's lucky pair of playoff underwear.

We didn't even come close to having enough equipment to use them as they were designed to be used. We were wiping down the entirety of disposable gowns and caps with chemical wipes so they could be reused if they were still in one piece, and we were sending the N95 masks to a sterilization center that the hospital had to create because we couldn't afford to throw the masks away. Each week Nurses were given extensions on how many times the masks could be sanitized before they were at the limit and no longer functional. The problem there was that since nobody knew anything about COVID, nobody knew the best way to treat it. The plan was to have maximum protection at all times against any sort of transmission: contact, droplet, airborne. We all looked like low budget astronaut cosplay characters.

There was a general understanding amongst those of us in the trenches that management was making it up as they went along. It was as if one hospital would hear what another hospital was doing and make *that* the ensuing week's policy. It filled our staff with a sense of disbelief, when the people who were supposed to have disaster management training at the highest level were putting the most ridiculous shit on display week after week after week. It was a living and breathing Catch-22 as we made extensive efforts to minimize our time in the rooms, however, these patients were so sick and would die so quickly that we were in the rooms nearly all shift anyway. We did things like keep IV poles with half-a-dozen or more medications hung on the outside of the rooms, running extension tubing from the pumps to the patients- Heaven & Earth help you if you got any air bubbles in the tubing. The management teams wouldn't show their faces on the ICU for fear of COVID-riddled air, yet some would shout out directions (over email or from some other safe distance) on how to reduce contamination. As if we all weren't swimming in that shit from the moment we stepped foot onto the Unit.

Looking back on it all, I'm baffled at the insanity of how cyclical our shifts were. Half the time, your patients were running fevers and sweating off all the equipment—reread Part 2 and add in these specialized neuro monitoring electrodes to ensure proper amounts of sedation, paralyzing medication effectiveness, even back to basics equipment like the clear sticky sheets that hold down IVs, the Nurses were constantly fixing to maintain the access needed to deliver the medications required to keep a person alive. Changing sheets underneath people so they wouldn't get moisture injuries. You would finish a task just in time to have one of your medication pumps alarm that it was about to run dry. At any given moment, one of our patients would start losing the fight and you would watch their oxygen saturation plummet. Then the team would go into the room and make efforts to regain control. Just to have one of the other problems you recently fixed become a problem again.

One of the worst things to happen that turned into something positive was when the hospital had to cancel all their scheduled surgeries. This meant that all surgical Nurses were looking for hours to work and many of them were brought up to the ICU in a role we called "Helping Hands." Their assistance was PIVOTAL in helping things run smoothly by running laps around the unit and simply replenishing things. But if you can imagine, the entirety of each unit was massively crowded. Two long hallways, 12-patient rooms on each side for 24 in total, and in the middle there were three separate nursing workstations we called Pods. Each Pod had four rooms on either side of it

I wish medical dramas were more realistic and showed how often people shit themselves. The prevalence of this occurrence is pretty unreal. The ER doesn't hold this issue with much regard, however from the moment a person is brought into the ICU, any given Nurse is tracking their bowel habits.

COVID is a large topic all on its own—how to take care of people in itself can be so infuriating, let alone a virus as unpredictable as this thing. Patients would (and still do) comb the internet for days searching for things that can be done to treat COVID and, subsequently, want to take such measures over the researched, Doctor recommended approach to fix the problem. In the realm of medicine, 2020-2022 was a blink of an eye and, at the time of writing this, COVID has been around for two years and the primary argument for not following the prescribed treatment plans for COVID is that it was rushed and hasn't been studied enough; most people going against the grain have an argument that is summed up with "we don't know." People won't take the vaccine because they "don't know what's in it" or they will refuse the infusions because they "don't know what's in it" or because they "don't know the long term effects" and so on. I can absolutely sympathize with people who have a concern for the unknown and unforeseen effects. Hospitals following trends too early like Plaquenil certainly did not help Nurses do their jobs.

Now, being skeptical is by and large a positive thing. It is what leads people to question things and seek out answers or a better means of doing something or they find entirely new answers to problems. The issue with the "we don't know" contingent when it comes to the last two years is that, by this point, we *do* know a lot. We do know that some podcast prescriptions include overdosing on vitamins, drinking piss and or bleach, misting hydrogen peroxide in their face, or nuking their intestinal ecosystem with a medication primarily prescribed to horses by veterinarians which is designed to eliminate worms from your gut. Again, I have no idea how someone made the connection between deworming and intestinal parasites and managing a respiratory virus. I will never in my life be clever or funny enough to come up with an appropriate analogy there. What we do know is that the home remedies have been proven to cause more harm than good. Unfortunately, there is no great defense against the hottest "do your own research" trend when patients quite literally went through the scientific process nearly as guinea pigs.

But people aren't going to do what they don't want to do. Even an "all hands on deck" approach to curbing a pandemic occurred for two years, and "we don't know" persisted because there is always more data needed. It is also disguised as faceless internet accounts of "I know somebody who got the vaccine and the next day they had a stroke" or vice versa where they have had COVID twice and it wasn't even as bad as allergies. COVID has been around for two years, tobacco has been around for centuries and there are still pockets of people who have used tobacco their whole life without problem so "clearly it is not the threat the industry wants you to believe it is."

But most people resistant to battling COVID fall into another group of people who think COVID brought about too little effect for how large of an inconvenience it is to perform or, even better, that efforts to manage a global threat are influenced by foreign enemies of the state. COVID really has ruined any future filmmaker's ability to believably write about a global threat. The film will immediately lose any credibility when they mention how the world united for a single cause.

This is the group of people that cry out, "I'd rather die on my feet than live on my knees! 'Murica!"

Let me tell you about those people. They don't die on their feet. They die belly up in a hospital bed with confused, oxygen starved brains after one to two weeks of moaning and groaning because they "don't feel good." They die with a tube in their throat shoving oxygen-concentrated air into their lungs, a tube in their stomach giving them liquid nutrition which leads to liquid shits, and that is if they're lucky enough to have liquid shits. Liquid shits means they get a tube docked at the end of their intestines to collect the liquid shit. If they somehow don't have skin burning acidic shits and have skin burning solid shits, guess what? Then their skin is harder to keep clean and they die with the adult version of diaper rash from laying in their own shit. Now, you probably read that thinking "Oh my God, those Nurses just let them lay in their own shit!" And the answer is no, not let them but at the same time when you're under staffed & have multiple unvaccinated future dead people to manage all at once, managing the multiple avenues of organ failure takes precedence over wiping someone's ass. And that is exactly what it is, wiping a full grown adult's ass for days on end like a little baby.

Back to it.

The arrogant and overly-confident die with a tube in their urethra, too (pee hole for the cheap seats) to track how shitty their kidneys are working. They die with arms that are more bruises than not and full of holes from IVs and monitoring devices because, when you are bloated, it makes it really difficult to get and to maintain an IV. They die sweaty and confused after days on end of frustration because they feel like crap because their kitchen sink modalities did not do shit. They die bloated, confused, gasping for air because of the progressive shutting down of all their organs

This book is ultimately about added complications of nursing. Added complications of COVID became doing the impossible for the ungrateful. Double digit hours of negotiating. And by "negotiating" I mean people refusing to do what they need to do in order to prevent the above scenario, people being persistent with their kitchen sink remedies despite their deteriorating condition. And honestly without being vaccinated it really isn't preventing, it's staving off. I said to myself, when I decided to take my collection of stories down the road of turning them into a book, that I would avoid any political bullshit but unfortunately the medical world has become one with politics. I can't tell you that unvaccinated people have ugly, miserable, drawn out deaths without 50% of the people that read this thinking, "This guy! Spreading his lies and agenda!" The same people that claim that getting vaccinated and wearing masks in crowded areas is allowing in the government too much but yet don't understand how ads on their cellphones work. I'm willing to bet most of them drive on the side of the road they're supposed to, wear seatbelts, have jobs, and I'm willing to bet they mostly abide by laws laid out by the government and recognize a good portion of civil structure—you know, some real, "living on your knees" things.

There are things that are done in the hospital that will assist a COVID-positive person with their oxygenation problem. We can increase the concentration of oxygen, the amount of volume delivered into the lungs, and the pressure at which the volume and/or higher concentration is delivered. You see, pulling air into your lungs is a process that is typically done with negative pressure—in a normal situation air is pulled into your lungs, it is not pushed in. But when your lungs are filled with any form of infection pulling that air in gets a little dicey. So to assist oxygen reaching its destination, the hospital uses devices to push it in or increase the amount in hopes that the increased amount will find its way through.

Neither of these means are particularly comfortable, especially the pressure. But it means life or death. It means life or death with that utter sincerity and stark contrast that the phrase 'life and death' holds. If you do this, you have a fighting chance—unvaccinated people's fight is less of a knock down, drag out fight and more of a one-on-one versus a mother bear protecting her cubs but there's still a chance things will work out. It does happen.

The obstacle again is discomfort. Believe me when I tell you that most people in this situation choose death. Read that again. Maybe a couple times. Now, of course I don't mean they choose death like they've been given the option from a classy restaurant menu and directly acknowledge it like, "Ah, yes. I see death is the staff's recommendation. I'll have that." I mean that the whole no pain free option is in full force.

Let's start with the less irritable means. It is called Heated High Flow. Take any medical show you have ever seen and picture a patient with the plastic tubing that is running between their upper lip and their nose. That strip of tubing has two prongs that fit inside each nostril and deliver a small amount of oxygen through each nostril into the respiratory system. A Heated High Flow device is that thing on steroids.

It is larger so it can deliver a high flow of oxygen into your nose for you to inhale into your lungs. You know the phrase, "Not out of the woods, yet"? Well, people with COVID that need this device are on the perimeter of the woods. They are either walking into the thick of it or are through the thick of it and entering the clearing once again. If things get dicier than what that device can handle, there are two other options that we will get into. Now, as I mentioned, this thing blasts oxygen into your nose—hence, the High Flow—the *Heated* part of the name comes from the fact that the air needs to be warmed up. At the base of the tubing there is literally that: a warmer. Actually, a more appropriate name would be Humidified Heated High Flow because the warmed air is flowing through a reservoir of water.

Typically, when you breathe in air the hair and folds on the inside of your nose will do a fine enough job of warming the air so it isn't irritating to the rest of you as it travels to the lungs. With this device, the blast is just too strong and blasts straight past these measures and does not give two shits about stopping for comfort. So, the warmer device attempts to make up for that. It does an okay job but still after a couple hours on this, it doesn't matter . . . that blast of air burns. It is like having a permanent sore throat in your nose. But the rub is that if you stop the device giving you air, you die. There is no if's or but's. You die. I promise you the Nurse, the Doctor, the respiratory therapist, none of these personnel are withholding a more comfortable means of saving you.

How aggressive the flow will blast *does* have a range and the percentage of oxygen that it can add to the flow of air can also be adjusted. The higher the flow required, the more irritating it is on the nose—pretty standard thing to understand there. The amount of oxygen does not have an effect on the person's comfort but it does have effects on your body that can make taking care of these patients more difficult—that is why patients receiving this treatment get their blood checked regularly to ensure it is still needed. However, this means more needle pokes which just sucks.

Next, the warmer on this device is not fitted with a control dial so that each patient can find their specific temperature for comfort—it isn't a smart mattress finding your best zone for sleep; your options are "warm, less warm, or off." And even then the intent behind the design is that various oxygen delivery pieces can be used by the patient and depending on which piece is attached would determine which of the two temperature settings the machine holds—it is just that through experience, I have learned that some people find one or the other set temperature more tolerable. Not comfortable but more tolerable. Or even more accurately: less uncomfortable. There may be a market for this dial temperature thing, hmm . . .

Anyway, this thing can go far but only so far. If a person is on high enough settings—a huge blast of air coupled with a high percentage of oxygen—and they are still not oxygenating well then, the next option is an oxygen mask attached to a machine with a multitude of features. It is called Bi-PAP for Bilevel Positive Air Pressure.

I was going to wait until the end of this part to tell readers that both of those devices are not strictly for COVID, and that they serve purpose for dozens of conditions. It isn't like they were created alongside the COVID vaccine or anything, but man alive, would I love to see some statistics on how much their uses have risen in the past two years. People literally have home devices that are a form of this mask. You see them all the time in movies.

The hospital grade ones, to recycle an analogy, are that mask but that mask is *juicing* (again, on steroids). It is made of hard, clear plastic, and fashioned into a rounded edge triangle sort of tent that sits over your mouth and nose like a facehugger alien. The ventilation tubing runs from the vent machine to the center of the mask. It has a harness that runs over the top of your head like a mo-hawk, a hinge point at your forehead where the apex of the mask can hinge and lift up. The harness runs over the top of the person's head and has a central point at the back of the head where a series of straps (that tighten around your head) join together. I have only ever seen ones with four straps: two running over each ear at the temples and two more running aligned with the jawbone on each side.

The point of all that is to make it tight on your face. This thing comes into the fold when a patient's lungs are junk to the point where they are not doing their job effectively at all. The lungs are to the point where, not only do they have way too much crud in them to perform an effective gas exchange, but hell, they can't even move the air into the lungs to get to that point. The modality is meant to force air into a person's lungs and use a ventilator to mimic an effective breathing pattern to the best of its ability. The force behind the machine is why the mask is designed the way it is.

I don't know if I have to spell it out that this thing is uncomfortable. It presses on your face and works relentlessly to change your breathing (for the better), it does this by pushing air in and maintaining some pressure, even when you exhale. It dries out a person's lips, tongue, and whole damn mouth. People are nearly impossible to hear with this thing running so communication is altered, and most Doctors will take away eating privileges because, at this step, you are one step away from being intubated—being sedated to the point of having a breathing tube in your windpipe—and having a stomach full of food can complicate that procedure. Liquids pass through your stomach much quicker so most Doctors are cool with you getting by on that, but not all.

You would think people that have reached this point would be too sick or too continuously exhausted to give a crap about being uncomfortable. And you would be wrong . . . so wrong. This is a pretty aggressive means of keeping a person from being intubated, or as we so lovingly say in critical care, from "buying a tube," but it increases the odds of success in the fight, especially if a person uses it early or even just a couple hours like while they are sleeping. This is a practice we try to do but I tell you what, the majority of the time people will wear it for a few minutes, sometimes an hour or so. If I am lucky, they will use their call light to tell me that they "just can't take it anymore" and then tell me that "Hey, they wore it for a little bit" which is 100% more hopeful than anything else. See, the thing is that changing a person's blood chemistry through oxygenation is technically faster using the respiratory system than the metabolic system, but here's the thing: When we want to check the true effectiveness of how a new means of delivering oxygen is working, we will draw blood after typically six hours or more from the change. Not 20 minutes.

Wearing that thing sucks and sucks hard, but again, nobody is *withholding* the less-shitty ways of getting better from anyone. But still, they are negotiating . . . oh, Lord, the negotiating. I inform a patient the same thing that I just ended the previous paragraph, that it takes time to see changes and without adequate time wearing the mask, they are essentially continuing the walk towards death. I say this because there is no point in trying to fluff, and there is no point in agreeing with them because, as their medical representation, if I were to nod and shrug my shoulders to give that "hey, yeah, maybe we *can* try something else" vibe, I am then doing a massive disservice to the patient and anyone that cares about them. The stark truth is the only way to go.

But yet, their near-consistent response to this isn't that of a soldier who rallied, and inside is screaming, "It is this or death, so let's fucking go and do this!" It is that of a caving will power. People make a crying face and throw a stammering temper tantrum, and you would think that they just helped clear Omaha Beach and I am asking them to get into a Higgins Boat for Round 2. They act like they have put in the world of effort and here I come, the asshole, asking them to do even more. They choose the comfortable death over the uncomfortable fight. It isn't with any sort of glee or humor that I write that. Trust me, it is out of frustration. And even saying that it is comfortable is a misnomer. It is an exhaustive, frightening, uncomfortable path that lasts days to sometimes weeks.

People get to where standing up at the side of their bed (so they can take a shit in a framework toilet called a Bedside Commode_ becomes taxing on their oxygen levels—to the point where they may not recover from it. They get to the point where literally any movement will send them into a coughing fit that lasts for an hour. All the while, negotiating continues until it literally can't anymore as COVID has stripped the option from them and that breathing tube is necessary to push air into their lungs, their bodies using every last calorie of energy to fight for more time.

And so what's a better representation of "problem behind the pain" than all of that? COVID created a new kind of problem for all of us, yes. But more than anything, it *exposed* a vast array of problems in our country and beyond—perhaps these problems stretched back for centuries and some chose to bubble up to the surface in the Year of Our Lord 2020. But as for the years ahead—be it ER or ICU or WTF—let's all take a moment to examine our own pain threshold, because the other side of it lies our fate. You may never experience a life-threatening bout of COVID-19, but we all experience downgrading health and the necessary medications/procedures to make us better. When (not "if") those times come in life, please please please remember this one thing: the people trying to hurt you are actually there to help. For the love of God, let them do their work, and dig deep down inside your pain threshold so your body can do yours.

PART 6: THE MODERN-DAY HOSPITAL

There's a decent percentage of people out there who have a general idea of how unruly taking care of another human being can be. Whether those people were raising children, caring for aging parents, or taking care of others in their profession.

In medicine there are specialty departments, specialty studies, specialties for everything. Areas that focus on every phase of life a person goes through are called speciality populations: young, old, bariatric, pregnant, etc. The discussion on how vast and specialized things get could be a series of books in itself. The ER, however, does not pick and choose, the ER is "come one come all". Our beloved elders (Silent Generation & Baby Boomers), the sandwich generations (Gen X & Millennials), and their kids (Gen Z). Each area has their own unique aspects that can deviate how an RN needs to approach managing their needs.

CHILDREN & ELDERLY

A brief generational overview isn't enough to explain the modern day hospital. Just like all the specialty areas an ER RN needs to study, like cardiac resuscitation, management of a trauma patient, blood clots, diabetic crises, etc. The ER RN has additional studies in how the body systems affect their patients over their lifespan. So when a Nurse sees the patient the patient they have just had assigned to their room is a child, the nursing brain switches to things to remember like how children's airways are different anatomically, how their vital signs would be different and to change the monitor into pediatric settings so it isn't falsely alarming over a heart rate of 120bpm. But just like all those hero stories of nursing, what the textbooks don't mention is that kids are tough.

Yup, the most important thing to remember going into that room is that kids can be tough.

Okay, the more accurate thing to say would be many kids' parents are tough and they raise tough kids. In essence, some kids suck because their parents suck. Now, I know there are plenty of "not tough" kids out there, I even know a few. Hell, I have even once or twice met some *nice* little kids. And I will also say that the bottom line on kids is that nobody, not a single soul, wants to see a sick or terrified kid. Now, from an anatomy standpoint, there are many different challenges a child might face. And from a *nursing* standpoint, when a child is sick, in a weird kind of way, our job gets easier because a sick kid doesn't fight getting help. They may initially be resistant but they don't fight when they are in an emergency. They don't toss the neck brace off and throw a fit because of how uncomfortable or boring the ER gets.

Of course, if they are ill but not emergent, their personality comes out a little more . . . placing the parenting on full display. In my time as an ER Nurse, I have met a megaton of unruly kids. Unruly because their parents are unruly, simple as that. It has absolutely nothing to do with the reason for their visit. Some have been sick, some have been extremely sick, while others had minor needs like Tylenol and Pedialyte. Kids have needs that span from emergent airway problems, appendices gone bad, to minor upset stomach management, to the bizarre mother who parades around with her child's snot-filled tissues.

But what makes these problems shitty is when we have to do our workup on the unruly child. Nearly all kids throw a fit, which is expected. As a child, adhering to any part of the plan in the ER—getting poked, examined or swabbed for samples —absolutely sucks. Even having a stranger look at a kid puts them on their heels. Think about how even full-grown adults act like they have never had a cold in their life when you come at them with a throat or nasal swab. Many adults legitimately whine, cry, move away, grab your arm, shove you away, give an exaggerated gag reflex . . . all sorts of childlike things. When adults act like everything that happens in the ER is the next worst thing that's ever happened to them, I can hardly put it past actual kiddos to do the same.

But what makes caring for kids less than ideal is damn near always a negotiation involved. Parents will also put Nurses on the hook for their bad parenting. They will promise that if the kid, for instance, takes the medication that the Doctor ordered, then a reward will follow. "If you do this, then the nice Nurse will give you a treat!" No, I won't. Why? Because the hospital isn't the County Fairgrounds and there is no stash of fidget spinners, crayons, or stuffed animals. The only treats we give is the gift of better health or at least provide the path to getting better.

In the negotiation process, parents either don't have the gumption to discipline their child or they don't want to be the bad guy. They want to be their friend or their pal. They don't like to get involved to the point where they make the visit difficult as all hell for Nurses. They tell the kid lies like, "It's candy!" then they follow up the statement by letting their kid taste a bit of the medication. Obviously, it *isn't* candy and, to the kid, it tastes like mid shelf cat urine. Even the children-targeted medications, which are less awful, certainly aren't on par with candy. The parent's lie becomes exposed and the Nurse ends up wearing the medication after the kid spits it out and their inner tantrum Spartan kicks down the chained doors that held it back.

After the candy strategy fails, Nurses will try an assortment of tricks but eventually end up wearing that medication as well. Some kids are lucky to get 50% of the dose down the hatch. And all the while Mr. & Mrs. Don't Discipline are sitting there . . . armchair quarterbacking the whole situation, saying infuriating things like, "I know this is no fun, we don't want to do this to you." The room quickly feels like an exorcism with the Nurse tossing the "healing stuff" at the possessed child flailing about in the ER bed with perpetual energy while the terrified parents are cowering and shakily trying to get the attention of the F-5 tornado equivalent of a miniature human.

Eventually, the parents are the ones that break, and can no longer take the situation at hand—they'll ask for the Nurse to come back after the child has had some time to calm down. Which is pretty agreeable because the Nurse likely has five other patients all wondering where the hell they have been. This is also where the negotiations truly begin but that doesn't affect me because it is typically things like, "We will go get ice cream after, you can watch your favorite show when we get home", and so on.

Many parents also want their kids to feel comfortable, so they let them terrorize the hospital room . . . which in turn leads to someone finding the Nurse assigned to the kid and reprimanding them for not parenting someone else's kid. But still, kids getting run over by a speeding gurney simply cannot happen so Nurses often have to parent someone else's kid. Just how it is.

Upon return, it is typically time to get the job done. Typically, the scenario is the child blanket burrito (swaddling). Not a single person leaves the scenario without a little bit of a guilty bully feeling but the fact remains that some children are not going to get better without it—an even worse situation would be letting the child's illness progress to the point where they feel so bad that they don't care. To reiterate, a truly sick kid does not care that much, if at all. It is actually an assessment note that healthcare providers make. If a child (who should be giving you "stranger danger" vibes) is nonchalant about a very unfamiliar situation, they are truly sick. It is a common sign to look for.

There is also a pattern in how the parents behave that will have a great effect on the child's behavior. And the point is certainly never going to be "Don't be afraid for your kids," it is simply informative. From the beginning, if the parent is frantic, the kid is going to freak out even more. Even under moments of high duress, when a child is indeed very sick, parents that are able to participate in the plan of care will help the staff through comforting their child as well as reinforcing the necessity of anything medical that needs to be done. The child intuitively returns to being calm after each interaction with the ER staff, which helps the overall process. If the parent is visibly displaying their nervousness, consistently reacting to intervene or playing the role of "protective friend" it is noticeable by the child and in turn breaks down cooperation.

To summarize a key point: The ER is definitely an area where a parent will learn a new depth of strength they themselves didn't know they had. Also, don't lie to your kids, folks. Just don't.

On the other end of life's spectrum, the elderly are either total badasses or a special form of "unable to handle discomfort." Think of how much you don't like things out of your daily routine and then add 40 to 50 years to reinforce your preferences. Add decades of wear-and-tear to degrade your body, reduce your tolerance to temperatures, add a stiffness to your bones and joints, which under the best circumstances require a longer warm up time than a diesel engine from the 70s just to get out of bed. In the ER, helping an elderly person with tasks that involve movement will have you well past "behind" on other patients' needs. Hell, your phone might even need an update.

In the nursing sense, it is a battle meeting their needs—they "gotta have their Oxy 10s every 4 hours" otherwise their situation is even more unbearable. There is no amount of warm blankets in the ZIP code to keep them warm. It makes for a lovely time when the patient has an IV medication ordered and the Nurse needs to sift through the entire south wall of JOANN Fabrics to find the IV.

There is a high likelihood that night shift Nurses will have one of two personalities with every elderly patient. They will have the daytime patient and the sundown patient. Sundowning is one of those mental decline cruelties that embodies the whole "truth is stranger than fiction" phrase. It is a horrifying situation that you don't wish upon anyone. Late in the day, a patient will be in their room, briefed on their workup, reassessed and vitals updated, then informed what the next aspect of the ER will be and how their next update should be in an hour or so. Everything will be agreeable.

Until . . . the Nurse is with their other patient for about 15 minutes and the Unit Clerk gives them a call because their previous patient is in a panic and climbing out of their bed because they need to get to their own wedding that happened in 1968. The situation is heart wrenching to behold. Patients that experience sundown will look you dead in the eye and tell you that the current year is 45 years prior. They will correctly identify their grown son or daughter in the room with them for who they are and in the next sentence state, with complete conclusiveness, that they are 25 years old and *really* need to get to that wedding. And all of that is after a 20 minute battle because they didn't remember you at all, and how you are a stranger breaking and entering their room at home.

A lot of progress can fly out the window, including their ability to be redirected back to the present. A particular danger is that, through confusion, things like infusing antibiotics or medications to control abnormal heart rhythms may get removed because the patient no longer remembers their purpose. Their risk of falling and sustaining an injury skyrockets and, to maintain safety, the patient generally requires person-sitting (like babysitting) to make sure the injury doesn't occur. Problem being, no ER has the staff to be able to pull that off. Emergency Rooms, as I've mentioned in this book, are chronically understaffed. The answer simply means more strain on an already-strained staff.

There is also a good chance these interactions will resemble a full moon rising on a werewolf.

These patients will string together some of the most offensive words that you can't even imagine. Slurs and insults that attack you in ways that you didn't even know you could be attacked. They will pick apart the obvious things that hate targets like your gender, skin color and/or body type and all its characteristics. Some might make a crass remark about your walk, your hair, your accessories, your accent, or your profession. They are capable of saying things that would make God go, "I made mankind but wow, I don't remember putting that feature in there." They will defend themselves to the death against a Nurse or CNA trying to get a set of vital signs. Just to eventually wake up in the morning, call you a 'dear' and ask if you would love to have some morning coffee with them. All with literally zero memory of who they were from dusk till dawn.

The latter of which falls into the "daytime" elderly patient which is typically sweet, kind, and patient. Which makes the werewolf version that much more sad. These are the instances where patient Nurses need patience . . . 100 fold. If you aren't, you might find yourself irrationally arguing with someone whose wedding took place 50 years ago. Take a deep breath, and know that none of us are outside of this phenomena sooner or later.

ALCOHOL, DRUGS, AND MENTAL HEALTH

By this point in the book, you might have a bone or two to pick with me which is fine—my intent for this book isn't across-the-board acclaim. If you read the title, you'd see I simply want a realistic portrayal of burnout and breakdown from an ER Nurse's perspective. With that being said, here is a brief paragraph about a serious topic before you read on. From this point forward, the book you hold is even less light-hearted. Writing on the frustrations of any given emergency scenario might, from a reader's perspective, rightfully carry some comedic value, and I've tried to convey some stories as such. However, things like booze, drugs, and mental health are pandemics for anyone afflicted with any combination of the trio—whether the addiction is a personal battle for you or for someone you care about, substance abuse is indeed a version of Hell on Earth. I also chose to talk about these three together because the relationship amongst them is undeniable. Yes, there is a toss of a coin chance that, for any given patient, the triage note will speak about what affliction has brought someone to the ER and also end with a casual, "patient also admits to methamphetamine use." But how many people treat their mental health crises with booze and street drugs is astoundingly depressing.

Alright then.

ALCOHOL *SHUDDER*

I've mentioned many stories throughout this book—not all of them speak to the universal ER, but some of them speak to universal truths. Alcoholics provide case studies of how those truths might fly out the window at any moment. And unfortunately, some Nurses whitewash the reality of what it is like to have a patient who's chief complaint is "Alcohol Intoxication."

Alcoholism is indeed a vicious addiction and is not a monster that goes away just because you close your eyes. To appropriately fight a monster, you have to become monstrous—just the way *it* is. The top tier of "worst human interactions" I have ever had in my life are all alcohol related, and I've been to Iraq.

I mean, consider the following. If a place where alcohol is *served* doesn't want you there because you have crossed the line and had too much . . . there is a problem. Intoxicated people become highly volatile, and every last one is a powder keg. It is just that some explode into crocodile tears and texts to exes but most explode into actual fits of rage and physical violence. And that is just interpersonal. Once you realize the danger that alcohol presents to a person medically, you will start to think that maybe prohibition wasn't that bad of an idea after all.

I mean every word and believe that alcohol, through any situation, is a fucking problem. Intoxicated people lose all sense of patience, respect, and common sense. Hell, they lose everything all the way down to bodily function. The word "drunk" might paint the picture in your brain of a staggering, stumbling buffoon with piss and/or shit soaking the legs of their pants and you would be absolutely correct in that visualization—it is, in fact, a regular occurrence even in the ER. A comedic vision of a heckler at a baseball game might even pop into the brain, but still, does that vision end with "and he sobered up and had a great rest of his day"? No, it ends with that hilarious heckler waking up the next day with dry mouth, vomit breath, booze odored body sweat, red eyes, and a dizzying headache that brings fresh vomit and sweat with the slightest movement of sitting up in bed.

But alcohol can also derail other bodily functions beyond expelled liquids. Like a person's brain function . . . no duh, right? Well, enough of the stuff will suppress a person's inherent drive to breath. Through the medical looking glass, alcohol has several layers of problems. On the front end, someone who is highly intoxicated faces threats of injury—their coordination is impaired and, concurrently, alcohol is a blood thinning agent. This means that it interferes with your blood's ability to clot. So, they even lose one of the body's most native functions for survival. Where alcoholism gets extra tricky is over extended periods of time. Alcohol is a substance called a "CNS Depressant." CNS meaning Central Nervous System. This label is telling you that it is your brain and spinal cord. If those sound like they are pretty big fucking deals, it's because they are pretty big fucking deals. Alcohol reduces your brain and spinal cord's ability to do their job. That alone is pretty scary to me.

Telling an alcoholic, while they're drunk, that they're an asshole would be as useless as yelling at your cat for making you go to the dentist. But, if I'm being honest, telling an alcoholic when they're *sober* that they're an asshole when they drink is definitely warranted. In fact, more often than not, *that* is an alcoholic's good pal—one who can tell it like it is so that said alcoholic might choose to pursue the necessary long-term help they need. I have never had a sober person show up to the ER and accuse *me* of being the one who pissed in *their* pants. Intoxicated patients often show up to the ER after being picked up by the police while on a three day bender, fight tooth-and-nail to leave then pass out . . . just to wake up several hours later, then not only get pissed off that they have to leave but also accuse the staff of spending their money and losing their belongings. Intoxicated people will go to war on that hill, too. They will literally have no memory of the previous 72 hours but accuse Nurses of stealing their items or money with more conviction than a lawyer with video evidence of a crime.

Everyone loves Einstein's definition of insanity: "Doing the same thing over and over again expecting different results." Emergency Room Nurses might say something different. Events in the emergency room can conjure up degrees of insanity that will change you. Enter a scenario where a father and daughter were struck by a drunk driver that was speeding down the wrong way on a divided highway. Four car crash victims in total, caused by two vehicles and a lone survivor. The father and daughter were killed instantly. The intoxicated driver lived long enough to crawl out and possibly even see the ambulance lights. The survivor was the driver's buddy, blood alcohol just south of four hundred and not a scratch on him. National trauma standards state that he cannot be cleared until he is sober and able to properly participate in an assessment to ensure the alcohol was not masking any injuries.

So now he has to stay in the ER until he is sober.

All due respect to Einstein, but you know what insanity is? The survivor in this scenario has no idea what happened, no idea his friend is dead and no idea they killed a father and daughter in the process. Of course, this is just an anecdote *speaking to* the insanity of it all. The insanity of which is also revealed in how Nurses have to babysit this guy like a child at daycare for the next 12-15 hours while he berates the entire

ER staff for not letting him go because he has to get home so he can sleep and go to work in the morning. Insanity hits fusion driven thrusters and torpedoes down that rabbit hole when, due to medical confidentiality, nobody is not allowed to tell this guy exactly what special type of shit he is because that would be revealing medical information about other people.

In my humble opinion, D.A.R.E. America should be run by Nurses. The program attempts to prevent children from drinking by essentially educating them for a week on how to obtain drugs and alcohol, followed up by a grand finale of having them witness the after effects of a car crash. Except it is this banged up car that was probably pulled from the nearby junk lot. There's no zing, no punch, and worst of all . . . no strategy in their approach. All D.A.R.E. America really does is tease the interest of drugs and alcohol into the minds of children.

What they need to do is parade those impressionable youths through a hospital where career alcoholics' skin color looks like they have been bathing in yellow highlighter liquid. What if children witnessed these patients thrashing about, restrained to a hospital bed because their brain has shriveled and doesn't function anymore? What if children saw what alcohol can do to a person's coordination and general livelihood? Their muscles are wasted away and their hair looks like dust bunnies were swept from the corner of the room and glued to their head because alcoholic appetites aren't exactly nutritious ones. Their bellies are bloated and covered in varicose veins because their livers are swollen and the effects of a dying liver put undue pressure on their abdominal circulation. Their liver is shot, so they are unable to process harmful waste products that occur in everyday processes. They need medication to maintain what is left of their liver and other medication to perform functions that the liver would otherwise do on its own. I wouldn't expect the medical terms of how alcohol poisons a person to land with a 10-year-old, but even one to two minutes face to face with the effect might create a core memory. So if anyone from D.A.R.E America is reading these words, consider this my job application. Perhaps we could team up on a new way forward to instill not so much a fear but an actual education into the dangers of alcoholism, and how to eliminate the allure of alcohol in the process.

Back to biology. Eliminating waste from your body happens almost entirely through three forms: breathing it out, pissing it out, or shitting it out. Alcoholic patients in the ER go from anger to confusion to damn-near asleep to more confusion and back to anger all over again—a rough way to spend a Saturday night. The medication they take to eliminate waste and preserve that 3% of processing power their brain has left? Well, one of the primary ways that works is by decreasing the body's absorption of ammonia, the effect—note: not *side* effect, the *intended* effect—is diarrhea, so they spend more time than any living thing (that isn't a pig) confused and rolling around in their own waste. If witnessing the sight wouldn't linger with America's children and persuade them later in life to moderate their drinking, then the smell would.

Emergency rooms have become de facto drunk tanks and acute rehab clinics. If you're ever in the emergency room and there is not a drug or alcohol related event in there somewhere, you've found a four-leafed clover. Go out and buy a lottery ticket after you leave said ER. There is nearly always an intoxicated person in one of the rooms, whether from a medical standpoint, (such as they were in an accident and now they are going to stay in the hospital or are simply too intoxicated to be safely sent home), or they are there *for* alcohol intoxication and need to be monitored to make sure their body doesn't shut down and seize on them. Or merely they are intoxicated on something to the point of crawling over walking and they need to metabolize. Every situation is an ugly one. Mostly because of how painfully these substances complicate every situation medically and emotionally.

Real quick, allow for a brief factoid that has significance as it relates to the ER drunk tank. We have talked about various forms of communicating in the hospital—one of the methods of communication is the PA system. The point of a PA system is to call the attention of individual people *or* the attention of all staff . . . alerting them to the development of an emergent scenario. It serves to bring together all types of resources to the same place in a single instant. There are many announcements that are universal such as "Code BLUE" and "Code RED" (not to be confused with the best Mountain Dew flavor out there) or "STROKE ALERT" and the never-fun "TRAUMA ALERT".

An unfortunate reality is that we also have codes to let people know of imminent danger. Sometimes they are specific like a code for a person with a gun or a weapon, but usually they are a general overhead warning that a patient is throwing punches. Each hospital has their own unique PA code and/or announcement, but it typically includes a color, a fictional character or a made-up Provider's name (i.e. "We need Paul Bunyan in the lobby. Paul Bunyan, please report immediately").

Many times intoxicated patients will be in a "waiting for sobriety" situation and want to leave, however, it has to be with a sober person PRESENT at the emergency room. This causes regular fights between patients and staff. The first thing out of the stupid hole in their face is, "This is America, I am an American, I have rights and you cannot do keep me against my will!"

And I do mean fights. Not arguments. The overall safety of the hospital staff, Nurses in particular, is constantly at risk whenever there are drunk people in the department ... so essentially always. Dealing with alcoholics like these on a daily basis makes you understand what good things prohibition could bring.

Every facility also has a "regular." One or a handful of patients that are there weekly or more. They typically show up obliterated and just need a warm place to sleep and some food in their belly. Typically not an issue but it becomes problematic when they also do the "cry wolf" scenario. If the ER is packed, which it typically is, they will claim chest pain. Remember in the initial pages when it was mentioned how some people claim to "know the secret" to bypassing the line? This is it and it is infuriating. It misallocates resources away from people who are legitimately in a crisis. On top of that, I would love to tell you that people take the Chest Pain chief complaint as a potential life threatening event 100 out of 100 times, but that would be a lie.

The regular shows up, typically with EMS, too. They usually call 9-1-1 after one too many. Outside of that what transpires beyond the ER walls, I cannot say. All I know is that the only time I have ever seen a regular sober is after they have slept in the ER for double digit hours. Legend has it that intoxicated people used to go to the Police Station to sober up but then something awful happened where a drunk tank patron died from choking on their vomit. They were intoxicated to the point where they were essentially paralyzed, their body tried to expel the offending substance and the person was lying on their back, too drunk for a coordinated effort to even roll over and save their airway.

So now, the standard measurement is if the person can walk. If a person is picked up by the police and they are too intoxicated to walk, they come to the ER. Nurses will often bait these patients off of the EMS stretcher right on out of the ER with a turkey sandwich. Shit, that is what people are after more often than not. Many battles have been fought over those turkey sammies.

Nurses don't need the instincts of an old weathered sailor to sense a storm about to make landfall whenever one of their patients is under the influence. These patients are VIOLENT. It is an unfortunate truth that staff safety has become one of the most highly discussed areas for improvement in the nursing world. Problem there is that all the discussion never seems to be around anything legitimate like safer staffing ratios. They usually involve how to implement some new policy on how the Nurses and techs can double their already doubled workload to manage the violence. There is an entire organization whose purpose is to reduce and manage risk within healthcare on a national level but yet while Nurse's are getting their asses beaten daily by angry patients, the focus of safety is always things like making sure there are no water bottles at the computer stations.

If you had to read that last sentence a couple times because it made such little sense, you would be correct in doing so. It is that ridiculous. Ground level surveys amongst Nurses will tell you that they are in constant concern for patient safety because they are stretched too thin and they are concerned for their own safety because of patient temperaments. But yet when these organizations come through for their surveys, the preparation is always "make sure you don't have food or drink outside the break room" or "make sure you know our hospital's mission statement and where the chemical data sheet is located."

I digress.

While the ugliness of alcohol is frustrating enough on a societal level, the ugliness of alcohol in the medical sense can be life threatening. Prolonged usage leads to more than a developed tolerance . . . tolerance leads to dependence. Alcohol changes how your brain functions by slowing it down and alters how your nervous system communicates within itself and the rest of a person's body. How much and how severe has a direct correlation with how much and how often a person drinks but the effects are masked as long as a person is drinking and the severity of the effects of alcohol can be very sneaky to detect.

After a person has had their last drink, the nervous system is not an easy thing to manage. Even as soon as 6 hours after drinking, they can develop mild symptoms like headaches, nausea/vomiting, tremors and restlessness. Think about that. Six is less than a standard work day. And for roughly 12 hours up to two days a person can experience hallucinations and seizures. In that timeframe up to several days later a person can become so severely confused that they become delirious, experience extremes in vital signs with a dizzyingly rapid heart rate, exhibit stroke-threateningly elevated blood pressures, and develop fevers to a life-threatening, seizure inducing level. These patients need extremely close monitoring for several days, often requiring an admission into the Intensive Care Unit.

And so, lest I offer you new story after story in the ways in which a "fun night out" can lead to a horrific night in (the ER), I will wind down with this: alcohol has its place in society, and alcohol unfortunately has its place in the ER room. If there is any hope in mitigating the latter, we need to examine the former with a mature lens. And how do we do that? Well, here's a brief exercise for you . . . put down this book, and go stand in front of the closest mirror you can find (probably somewhere in your home). But don't just stand in front of it. *Look.* Look really close at the person you see. That person was once-upon-a-time the child who was being told such dangers of alcohol. Maybe *you* were the kid sitting criss-cross-applesauce at a D.A.R.E. America presentation, swearing you'd never drink alcohol . . . until you actually did in high school just a few years after the fact.

No matter where you fall on the alcoholic spectrum—from never having a drop to "Houston, we have a problem."—that person in the mirror has the capability to get help ASAP *or* support someone else so they can get help. Progress may not happen right away, but in the months and years ahead . . . the average American emergency room will thank you for it.

DRUGS

There's another set of substances many children swore off in elementary school only to "dabble" shortly thereafter. "Altered Mental Status" is typically the chief complaint for a person on drugs. Maybe it is simply because there are way too damn many drugs out there for it to get its own check in title whereas it is a safe assumption that "alcohol intoxication" isn't in reference to a person chugging a bottle of isopropyl or rubbing alcohol. The amount of illicit or prescription drugs a person can get their hands on is astounding. When it comes to drugs versus alcohol, some wonder if one is particularly better than the other. Maybe, maybe not, but let me tell you from my frontline experience: alcoholics are way more violent and difficult to deal with. People that have an addiction to drugs are usually way more honest about it, too. Maybe since alcohol is legal, people aren't as ready to see it as a problem? Who knows . . .

Yes, there are violent people on drugs and yes. On the flipside, I have had some extremely polite alcoholic patients, legitimately some real "salt of the Earth" types; rarely is anything in medicine consistent like gravity. But there is a relatively large population of people on drugs who are too busy hallucinating and, oftentimes, they are *scared* not only in the moment of being high but when they come down as well. There is also a chance that whatever drug the person is on is one that has them euphoric or simply too zoned out to be a raging bull. Unfortunately, one of the fan favorites is Methamphetamines. Meth is some violent shit, no doubt, when a patient on drugs becomes violent, they are violent with the strength of ten men, it's insane and they are a nightmare to have as a patient but for reading purposes, to describe any violent person on any brand of drugs you could just read the alcohol section and replace every "booze" reference with the offending street drug reference.

Again, D.A.R.E America should show *these* people to the impressionable youth. Witnessing a person terrified and unsure of what is real or not for hours on end with no choice but to ride out the storm would likely leave an impact. Witnessing a person enter a dissociative state and thrash about like a cornered animal or those doing the cornering would imprint a core memory. Difficulties in having a patient out of their mind on drugs presents similar challenges as alcohol, with a handful of detail changes. The first is a 50/50 chance their families are in complete and utter denial that their son or daughter or whoever would do drugs in the first place. It's those family members (as opposed to the patient!) who let the Nurse know It's going to be a long night. Combating a family member's interjections, for several hours on end, while the hospital is humming is a recipe for hours of tension.

In terms of the *severity* of one's addiction, a patient will deny to the best of their ability, which makes for some dark comedy in its finest form. The conversation typically looks like this:

"I *do* use drugs, but only weed. And occasionally heroin. But that is only when my cousin comes to town."

"I see. And does your cousin come to town often?"

"She lives in the next town over . . . "

"Okay, so safe to say weed and heroin are the culprits here."

"Well, weed is for sure, but only sometimes heroin. If I have the money I'll do cocaine. If not, then just meth . . . but that is only when my cousin comes with her friends because they like meth and I don't want to be a bad host."

By the end of it, the Nurse and patient might as well be in a confessional booth with the list consisting of weed, edibles, ecstasy, cocaine, heroin, meth, PCP, acid, mushrooms, Xanax, valium, pain pills, ketamine . . . a list that is far from exhaustive.

My advice, from the inside of an ER environment, is that if you are a family member of someone on drugs and have a hand in helping them to the ER: Pack it up and go home after they're there. Sure, call in once in a while to see how he or she is doing. But I say "keep your ass at home" because, otherwise, you are in for a long, *deep breath and exhale* LONG (like "longest night of your life") sort of night. People having a bad experience while on drugs deal with it for several hours. And thanks to a general public that is educated through only news headlines and social media, people are overly sympathetic and equally stupid when it comes to confusing heroin with mental illness. They sit there at the patient's bedside and get worked up all night long because they don't understand why their loved one is wigging out on meth, and are utterly convinced that they are having a psychotic break.

It's quite detrimental to witness someone you care about have a bad trip. Those friends and/or family members under the influence become worried, anxious, fearful, and sometimes hallucinate and act out in erratic behavior for several hours. The entire time, minutes seem to pass like hours and the family member is growing impatient and frustrated that "nothing is being done." When a family member makes the awful decision to ride this day or two stretch out with the person, it sucks for them, it sucks for the Nurse, it sucks for everyone involved—so it goes with any addiction-ridden family (which, for the umpteenth time, is far too common in America because we are broken humans who glorify the things that break us).

In such a case, Nurses are bombarded with the same requests while we're just trying to care for their loved ones in the best way we can. What people need to know is that the point of their loved one's stay in the ER is to make sure they are safe.

During that time, which certainly can take days, we look out for heart issues, breathing issues, fevers, which are all those pesky things called putting a plan together, we monitor for detrimental effects of withdrawal. People hallucinating will do some wacky shit, like exclaiming how spiders are coming through the floor to pull them under the crust of the Earth, claim that invisible people are using their minds to electrify them or whatever assortment of bizarre occurrences, but unless there is a problem that needs to be addressed to immediately save the person or keep them from running wild, the antidote is time . . . and lots of it. Under severe circumstances, knockout drugs and a breathing tube. Everyone is so utterly convinced that those bizarre behaviors must be due to mental illness because a friend of a friend of one of their Aunts responded to their Facebook post about how they need to have the person examined for mental illness.

There is a direct correlation between mental illness and drug abuse, yes. But that is what it is, a *correlation*. It's not causality. But let me throw this grade school exercise at you to clear up the point.

Consider the following elementary school logic conundrum:

True or False—If all lions are cats, then all cats are lions.

It's false and we all know it. So, let me rewrite the problem by inserting an Emergency Room scenario.

True or False—If all people with mental illness do drugs, then all people who do drugs have mental illness.

Also false! And if you didn't consider it by now in life, I hope you take that reality to heart. This means that your typically sweet friend or family member, free from any mental illness or diagnosis, that is doing whackadoo shit when they have never done whackadoo shit before in the strongest of likelihood does not have mental illness.

Now is an appropriate time to remind you I certainly do not know all there is to know about mental illness, but I *do* know that people, especially young adults, tend to have psychotic breaks in their late teens through their twenties and that stress can influence this i.e. college stressors, job hunting, etc. And in this economy? I mean . . . What *doesn't* stress people out anymore?

That being said, I stand by my statement that many patients have likely deviated from the straight and narrow to try enough substances that would win Blackout BINGO. Who could possibly know what crazy shit is out there and will be making headlines tomorrow? Hell, the lengths people will go to in order to get high has NASA level ingenuity. Remember bath salts turning people into flesh eating zombies? If not, look up Jenkem to see the lengths people will go. And if that doesn't make you want to donate to your local anti drug campaign, Krokodil might. There is certainly a larger issue to talk about when discussing drugs and the problem they are. I believe the best format to bring the worlds of the large-scale drug problem and Emergency Nursing is how conversations with Nurses seem to talk about regions of the country and their pairing drug problems like it is a badge of honor. RNs will try and out compete each other for the bullshit they've endured through conversations such as "Oh you think your state is bad? Mine is the meth capital of the country!" It's frustrating that some take pride in the fact that one's hometown has more heroin overdoses per capita than any three other states combined.

So, to summarize, don't hang around the ER for 10 hours and have a mini coronary every time they act differently than you have ever seen before. They are operating on *drugs*. Nurses in the "psychological hold" area of an ER have three to four other people doing the same thing. Go home—don't blemish the memory you have of this person that you care about by seeing them act possessed and ask the same three questions every 30 to 60 seconds for 12 hours. Don't be a helicopter parent to your 34 year-old drug addict. It's *our* job to get your son or daughter back to normal. It's your job to love them through the pain and know they're not the only one suffering in this way. And maybe reinforce to them that drugs are bad.

MENTAL HEALTH

To say the United States of America has a mental health problem, as it relates to the healthcare system, is possibly the largest understatement written in this book.

This country desperately needs more funding for its psychological hospitals. Or maybe the development of ERs that center around psych-specific matters is more accurate to say. While it is not my preferred patient demographic to work alongside, it *is* an area (when given the opportunity) where I feel like I am helping people in a difficult situation. And that help extends beyond the patient. Nurses assist these families in a difficult season of life and that shit feels good—like you're truly making a difference. For as many suicidal and nightmarish-type scenarios we see on a regular basis, there are just as many cold and hungry homeless individuals that come waltzing through our ER doors. In each instance, we try to help individuals accordingly—even if it means pointing them to another place or resource where they may receive better help than what we could provide.

Working the mental health aspect of emergency is under the same roof as the trauma bays, yes, but is a different beast entirely—I've seen Nurses have patients that survived a suicide attempt by chasing a bottle of Tylenol down with a bottle of Gorilla Glue, who then ran a spool of Duct Tape around their head to seal the deal (and yet somehow survive the process). Another who claimed to inject an entire syringe of antifreeze directly into their neck, which, apparently, only has one side effect and it is that it will turn someone into a raging jackass for 10-12 hours. Here is what I know to be empirically true in regard to psychological issues any patient might have: these "issues" might be *giving* patients a hard time, but the patients themselves are *enduring* through a hard time. And just like everything else mentioned so far, the path to getting better does not take a trip through Candy Land—it typically takes a guide (Nurse) and support system (patient family and friends) to reach one's final destination.

And when I say "patient family and friends" I do mean patience as in the quality our country would do well to promote more regularly. Enter the Emergency Room "Hold" period. Some people have heard of the term '72-hr hold' but have a misconception about what it means or the various types of holds. Many patients arrive and have a version of the phrase, "So what, now I have to sit in this room for three days?" The short and non comprehensive answer is . . . maybe. However, with Psych-related patients (which typically entail patients with psychological-related needs and/or specific requests) holds as opposed to medical holds, it most certainly does not mean that a person is on lockdown in the ER for a set time period of three days; in a way it really is the other way around. The idea is that when a patient checks into the ER for a psychological illness they need to be seen by a specialist. Just like a patient with a cardiac event severe enough might need to see a Cardiologist, or a neurological complaint, a Neurologist, a urinary complaint, a Urologist, you get the point.

Yes, there are some legal holds where a Doctor will not allow a person to leave the hospital for a designated amount of time. These holds are typically substance overdose holds and designed to keep a person safe from complications of experiencing withdrawal. It is to keep a person surrounded by personnel and medications to manage the situation should it become an emergency. Many of the times it is fine, the person simply feels a various level of hungover and annoys the shit out of their Nurse for three days asking for a sandwich and pudding every 90 minutes. But every now and then a person's vital organs don't like the fact that they have been treated like a punching bag and have issues with the recovery. Things like seizures and heart attacks can happen as the substance runs its course.

For mental health chief complaints, the wait can go from long and annoying to downright absurd. Think 24-full hours-or-longer kind of absurd. This is because the evaluator needs to do their assessment with the person in their uninfluenced mental/psychological state—free of drugs and/or alcohol that could be muddying the evaluation. And if there was ever a stronger marriage than mental health and home remedies of things like drugs and alcohol, I have yet to meet it. For patients that arrive with a mental health complaint, the psych professional won't even consider evaluating them until there is proof of sobriety. A breath or blood alcohol level needs to be documented and a urine toxicology screen has to be resulted. They also need to be medically cleared for the same reason.

Facilities are already strained enough, so the last thing they want is to go through the process of taking on a patient just to learn that the reason the patient thought their beard hairs were wires woven through their face as a punishment by God wasn't due to acute mental psychosis. It was meth. Or that the patient recycling his own urine because they thought they figured out that everyone's own body is the fountain of youth . . . was again meth and *not* schizophrenia. Or the patient that believed factions of the government had caught up to him and were electrifying his bed for things he did as a teenager, was in fact once more . . . just meth.

Now, with drug screening comes a divide which seems to be evaluator specific. If the provided urine drug screen shows any substance in it, the evaluator will wait for 12-24 hours to ensure sobriety before they are evaluated. There is a difference in some evaluator mindsets: some say they will run that clock from the time the person checked into the ER, because unless something went totally off the rails, the patient obviously did not shoot up while in their hospital room. Others will say that they have to have 12-hours from the resulting toxicology screening. It is probably at a higher level than anything at the bedside. It is probably a specific company rule.

Whenever I work in the psych section of the ER, the most commonly fielded question is "When will I be evaluated?" To which I say "I . . . am not sure." Because the Nurse that is at bedside, is typically not clued in, and we don't want to promise them otherwise. I have literally had an evaluator sitting FOUR FEET behind me with a paranoid schizophrenic patient wandering out of her room every 5-10 minutes for several hours just to ask me when their evaluation will take place and the evaluator did not so much as remove her eyes from her computer to tell the patient that I, the RN, was not in control of such a process—outside of sending the damn piss sample to the lab to be tested for drugs.

When it comes to emergency room psych patients, the RN basically passes out lunch boxes, blankets, and stands at the ready for war when the patient decides the wait is too long and they want to bulldoze their way to freedom. Through nearly a decade of having half a dozen or so of these patients each week, never one single time has the Physician placed preemptive med orders. Even when the patient has checked in for aggressive behavior. It is not uncommon for patients to be brought to the ER as a result of a violent situation. They will be aggressive towards everyone they meet, and the Physician won't even be able to get through their examination because of how violent, aggressive, inappropriate, etc. the patient is behaving.

What happens? Nothing. The Physician walks away because nothing says I'm not going to cooperate with you quite like answering questions with "Fuck you" or "Come near me and I'll kill you." In most places it makes sense to let the aggressive person be and give them time to cool down, but it's the hospital where *nothing* happens that is the problem. Nothing happens. The RN is left alone to sit there and stare at the angry patient for multiple hours while nothing happens before eventually deciding to take matters into their own hands. No amount of turkey sandwiches in the world will be enough to prevent this, I promise.

This is a heavily complicated situation, because once a patient is on a legal hold, they are not allowed to leave the ER. The only option is to call reinforcements. This is where the nursing staff will put on another one of those hats they didn't know they'd be wearing while in nursing school. And this head is more of MMA headgear. The person isn't legally allowed to leave and ends up getting dog-piled by the Nurses, ER techs, and security personnel and placed into restraining devices until the Physician can determine if the best route moving forward is to medicate the raging bull into a slumber. The problem is that the department absolutely cannot have a violent patient on the loose as they are a threat to not only themselves, but staff, and most importantly other patients. So, an ugly truth is that restraints are oftentimes a necessary evil.

However, once the situation has come to that, the plan immediately becomes to remove the restraints literally as soon as possible. Patients are at great risk of injury while in restraints so the patient is given a dedicated Nurse to monitor them until the situation calms down—usually until the medications kick in—and a pharmaceutical "sun's getting real low big guy" type of scenario ensues. Frustratingly, if the aggression boils to that point, it pauses the clock on a patient being evaluated. See, the mental health consultation is not allowed to take place if a patient is in restraints. They are actually supposed to wait a designated amount of time, typically four hours after an event to ensure that the patient is no longer aggressive or overly medicated.

There *are* slight differences among states, facilities, etc, but it mostly goes like this: if a patient has been seen by the emergency psych evaluator and deemed they cannot be safely sent back on their way, they then need to be placed in a short term facility to better straighten out whatever is ailing them. Now, if within 72 hrs no psych facility has accepted the patient for whatever reason—the usual reasons being capacity or a history of violence—they then have to be reevaluated by the emergency team to determine if they are still a threat to their own self or other people or if they are still what is called "gravely disabled." Gravely disabled is where a person's condition is so severe they aren't able to function and take care of themselves. It certainly is a definition that casts a wide net, I mean, every other person's coffee mug has some funny little print on it of how they cannot function until the coffee is below a certain line. Half the time I am inclined to believe their mug.

There are instances, from time to time, in which a patient will be in the ER for the full 72 hrs, however, during that time they have adjusted to the medications provided by the ER well enough to be safe to continue outpatient care and are then sent home. It is rare but it does happen. Most psych patients are typically agreeable to this. They have been dealing with their diagnosis for long enough that they have been through this ordeal and they have established Doctors, medications, lifestyle, etc. that helps them live an independent life. It is just that sometimes just like a person's physical body can have a momentary breakdown, a person's mental health just gets away from them and they need a hospital stay for a day or two. A lot of psych medications come with the side effect of drowsiness. We're talking "hit you with a tranquilizer dart" drowsy, too.

Facilities made with the purpose of addressing mental health are at crisis levels of being overworked just like the ER. Since they are a specialty aspect of health that the ER is referring to, they can usually set strict guidelines for acceptance: a typical reason patients don't get accepted at a facility is aggression. No hospital wants to take a patient that has a history—new or established—of violence. Violence is without a doubt a massive problem within the ER, but ERs don't turn away patients, even the violent ones. They just have to call reinforcements in the form of personnel and/or medications to manage the patient until their plan moves forward. With that, there is a fine line that is becoming invisible between mental health diagnoses and extremes in normal emotions.

People seem to be getting pushed over the edge into mental health crises more and more regularly, at home when your 12-year-old pisses you off and is behaving badly, don't depend on the ED to parent. Don't bring that preteen into the department claiming they need to be evaluated by a Psychiatrist then jet. And trust me, it happens more than a normal person would like to accept.

The common reasoning for parents bringing their kid(s) into the ER is typical kid issues like the fact that they don't want to clean their room or they don't want to finish their dinner. There was even one particular child (who will one day have some real mental health issues, I guarantee it) that was well known to all the staff at this particular hospital. He was just in a situation with a bad parent-and as a non-parent, I don't say that lightly. His mother would bring him to the ER usually at least weekly for similar reasons to those at the start of this paragraph. He very legitimately had been seen and evaluated by all types of medical specialties: emergency, neurological, psychological, etc in search of an explanation for any behaviors. And they all agreed that he was not in their wheelhouse and the consensus was that if anything at all he needed anger management. His mother brought him in so regularly that he had his own personalized special operating procedure, security would be notified of his arrival, he would get a dose of Benadryl and be sent home, a Do Not Pass Go sort of deal. The security became as much for his mother as for him. He was a terror and his mom would need to be kept from leaving as that was her M.O., drop off the kid then not answer the phone for a week—no joke, a week or so. Typing up a room that could be given to a person in a life or death mental health crisis.

When parenting calls on you to be a disciplinarian, be one. Parents cannot always play the friend or entertainer. If you deflect every time your kid misbehaves, it's only going to escalate. Which is a good word to end this whole section on alcohol, drugs, and mental health: deflect. The longer any individual deflects these problems onto the next day (and the next day and the next) the worse it will get over time, just like a cancer.

And the longer we, as a society, deflect from addressing these issues accordingly, we will only continue to spiral out of control. There will be more chaos and more civil unrest because we deflect the true issues that lead to self medication in the form of alcohol or drug abuse—both of which can lead to some serious mental health crises with lasting effects. I think there is hope, even if it's a slim chance. But the modern day hospital simply can't wait any longer for change. It was part of the reason I wanted to write this book—I know I can't change the system as a whole, but if I could help others think about these things just a *little* bit differently, then maybe all this typing was worth it.

PART 7: REPEAT

The system is too massive to handle large directional changes, but small steps of improvement could build up to necessary changes in the American healthcare system. So, it may seem picky but part of the change needs to include an important shift in vernacular: stop saying that "nursing is a calling." It is a job. Nightly, I will have patients say something within a couple degrees of that phrase, "it takes a special person to do what you do" and what is running through my mind every time is, "it takes a special person tell patients that they cannot have a drink of water somewhere between one and two hundred times a night? Yeah, I can see it but I don't think we both have the same 'special person' in mind."

Of course, that's downplaying the profession but there are absolutely nights when getting pain in the number of times someone asks me for water would garnish a higher paycheck.

The "calling" mindset reinforces that it's okay to work with unsafe nursing ratios and pending assault and abuse by patients and coworkers (other Nurses, Physicians alike)—all for a wage that is barely enough to pay the bills in most states. Nursing isn't a calling, but it also shouldn't be barely better than self-flagellation with no praise while simply waiting for Nurse Appreciation Week every year and ensuing social media posts of encouragement. That *joyous* week is also the week where certain hospital staff out there find a way to cut (normally 10 slice) large pizzas into 18 for everyone and take great pleasure in displaying a new T-Shirt design with the latest slap in the face word play like "We can't MASK our appreciation for you so we'll put it on a shirt" design. Available for convenient purchase by taking the $30 out of your next paycheck. Anyone who loves that "nursing is a calling" phrase is likely on the outside looking in, or they read some of those books I read years ago that paint it in a lovely light. Nursing, in all actuality, is a gritty and largely thankless job.

Nursing is trying to help people while fighting a battle on many fronts. Yeah, humans can be awful, and I've obviously spent a page or two in this book denoting that thought. But any problem begins with *recognition* of a problem. An early step in battling problems is education and prevention. Why do Nurses repeat the vocational version of slamming their head against the wall week after week? Honestly, the answer is probably amnesia. A whopping 99 out of 100 patients (give or take a few) leave Nurses wringing their hands raw with frustration, but for whatever reason, that *one patient* who expresses appreciation, is genuinely grateful, and works with Nurses to begin the healing process for whatever brought them to the ER, does seem to resurface the nursing school desire to help and washes over the previous 99.

A recent law passed pertaining to transparency in hospital pricing is a massive step forward, however, it is not being enforced in all hospitals. The awareness over such laws is nowhere near what it should be, because if people knew they could make a change, it might actually happen in some cities. For example, insulin shouldn't cost $30 a unit. That kind of shit is criminal to the point where *ground level* criminals would look at the financial breakdown and say, "Damn, dude. That's fucked up. I'll take your phone and cash but at least I'm not ruining you for the rest of your life"

The American public struggles because the American public isn't informed. Or, like a wonderful quote from the fictional figurehead Ray Zalinsky, *"What the American public doesn't know is what makes them the American public."* In addition to general awareness, the American public isn't educated. I love to educate patients and give them something of a foothold for future endeavors for better health. These handful of pages are just the tip of the iceberg with what I do. And honestly, I think that is an aspect that should transcend all jobs. Whenever I go to the mechanic, I would love to have a rundown of what they did, why they did it and things I can do to get the most out of my vehicle and prevent a multi-thousand dollar surprise. I would also love to read a version of what I've written for other professions—could you imagine all the "underbelly" things that say teachers or waste management employees see?

Now, I am not here to try and have nursing viewed as some sort of martyrdom, because there are hospitals where nursing is great and I am grateful for many of the opportunities nursing has afforded me. I have met some inspiring people like the lady who told me stories from the 1940s about bonding with other women while welding together airplanes for the war effort.

One last reiteration: being sick sucks, being hurt sucks, fear of the unknown sucks, and sometimes even *having* answers sucks. Imagine not feeling well and then going to the ER only to learn you have cancer. Nurses have to contend with all of these emotions but keep the pace of an ER room in the process. This is why I made that jab about having a bridge program so that Nurses earn a degree in Psychiatry sometime in their career. But really, I think there should be something to it where just by working you could earn credits toward a different profession because burnout is real. Terrifyingly real. And making your way through one time is hard enough but after a couple of years of ugliness when the "calling" of being a Nurse is revealed to be just another ugly job, you feel like your only option is to push through.

Imagine a job where, between 10 to 15 times a night, you have to not only deliver bad news to people but also be their emotional outlet and sponge up all their fear, anxiety, anger, and distress so that way you can work with them and do what needs to be done to quite literally save their life. Because even though aspects of a Nurse's job need to be done to subvert further disaster, Nurses still cannot do it without patient consent and as was written about earlier, people will hold back on necessary, sometimes life saving procedures because they aren't in the right headspace yet. Reasons like this are places that Nurses would love to have more time. Most Nurses go into ER work so they can be there for people in their worst moments, but get stressed out by the job because, somewhere along the way, it became a slog of 90 percent managing paperwork issues, political issues, CYA double and triple charting to 10% patient care. Which even half of that could be done through primary care. Starting to see why this section of the book is called Repeat?

PART 7: REPEAT

For this and many other reasons, Nurses (and especially those in the ER) develop a cutthroat business attitude. Now, I am not saying that a Nurse will violate your rights or be overtly disrespectful of your fears, but there is a job that needs to be done and ER Nurses are receiving pushback with every aspect of trying to perform that job. Even the empathetic ones, at least if they don't then they typically don't survive in the ER. The problem is that Nurses in the ER get so much shit thrown at them on an hourly basis, shift after shift, week after week, and so on, that having thick skin is absolutely necessary. If a Nurse lets the near-constant difficulty and pushback of the job break their stride, that doesn't stop the ER from moving. They *have* to catch up. If you break even for a moment, you have to rebuild that resistance needed to accomplish the job.

There are numerous issues that contribute to the overall complicated state of our current Emergency Room crowding. Hell, just merely mentioning the U.S. Healthcare system will automatically stir up an assortment of negative feelings. Initial scratches of the iceberg include things like poverty and socio-economic issues, access to healthcare for millions, education on things like first aid, the opioid crisis and over-prescribing, improper treatment and evolving treatment of substance abuse and mental illness, corporate greed, and (astoundingly enough) 2020 through present being the years of misinformation, which is one of the largest obstacles to providing care to people.

This book is not about laying the groundwork to all of these fixing issues, it is simply a perspective from the point of view of someone who has quite literally been face-to-face with the mixture of all these issues. I kept the perspective as "ground level" for two main reasons:

WE'RE HUMAN

The first reason I kept the contents of this book fairly informal and baseline is for the possibility of a real human-to-human connection, and to have a closer look at some of the things that are issues with every emergency Nurse on every shift. Even if that emotional response to reading everything was "Well maybe this guy should just consider a career change."

Trust me, I very much understand that most situations in the ER are the summation of larger issues—issues that require systematic change where change even can be made. But the fact remains that my experiences are a nightly reality, and it doesn't matter if there is an academic, political, systemic, etc. root cause. Also, my experiences are mine alone but certainly not isolated. A rough number from the Bureau of Labor Statistics website on how many of the 3.8 million RNs in the whole workforce work in an actual hospital (it doesn't break down by specialty within the hospital) is 1.7 million. So, take what you have just read and think about how there are 1.7 million other people out there with their own unique compilation of experiences detailing unfathomable ways humans have treated them . . . 40hrs a week . . . every week . . . repeat. Write into any search engine about the current and projected future of nursing and you will see that Nurses are currently leaving the profession in droves, and the ones that are sticking around are moving on from the bedside.

And *that* in itself begs the question: where do we go from here? If that question sounds familiar to you, it's because that question is on the back cover of this book.

That "we" in the question is for all kinds of audiences to ponder. In other words, "Where do Nurses go from here?"

but also "Where do Doctors go from here?" and "Where do patients go from here?" If you've stepped foot inside a hospital before (which is fairly inevitable for everyone) it's worth asking *yourself* that question because our actions are the only ones we're truly responsible for. How we answer that question of where we'll go from here might be more crucial to "fixing the healthcare system" than we might think.

WE'RE FALLIBLE

The second reason for writing this book from a "boots on the ground" level is that I have not personally worked in research. At least not yet, I would like to get involved but as for now, I don't have a first hand account as I do with Emergency Nursing. I can regurgitate nursing articles or provide cliff notes on countless healthcare headlines across multiple news sources, but in the end all that does is stack up numbers in your mind. Numbers that will jettison from your short term memory just like you were cramming for that quiz you put off in favor of seeing the latest movie release back in the day. I could rattle off the latest articles in leading Psychology journals that outline the correlation of high acuity situations with certain emotions which lead to a number of predictable displays of behavior. Or I could tell you how nursing conditions lead to staffing shortages and how staffing shortages lead to things like hospitals potentially (and/or prematurely) discharging patients home because there are no Nurses to take care of them and how that leads to poorer care and higher likelihood of readmittance . . . blah, blah, blah. That sentence reads and you might think, "Oh wow, that's bad" but would likely forget the true impact of this reality as soon as you bring your mug of coffee to your face.

On the other hand, if I tell you that I have more than once taken on the task of cleaning out months of layered dirt, broken down tissue, and maggots from an infected foot that was wrapped in dirty dish towels and grocery bags as a makeshift bandage because the person didn't have proper access to healthcare, it sticks with you past the delightful aroma from your mug of coffee. If I tell you things like obesity have risen X percentage and thus straining healthcare operations by X percent because of the numerous complications, it doesn't stick with you. Now, if I told you when people get sick, they generally get weaker, much weaker and obesity is problematic to the point where Nurses have found things like discarded wrappers and small dead animals in large peoples' skin folds because they were too weak to clean themselves for weeks on end, it paints a better (but still not pretty) picture for you, the reader. Unfortunately (maybe), there is no amount of vocabulary that can adequately affect your sense of smell when reading about things like a gastrointestinal bleed, where blood in a person's GI tract gets digested and passed out of a person the way normal waste does. They don't exactly make blood or feces scented living room candles. They certainly wouldn't make a blood AND feces scent.

I also didn't want to write something that might evoke strong emotions while missing the mark because every section was littered with twenty-seven references to works cited on the topic. In other words, Nurses get to where they are because they want to help others, but eventually leave in droves (like we're seeing in a post-2020 world) because of the revolving door of poor conditions. A main idea for this book was to suggest there are dozens of things that make the job much more complicated than it needs to be—whether it be unrealistic expectations of what the ER does for patients, or the ridiculous divide within the hospital and how management feels the job should be done (which might or might not actually happen that way), or how a large part of nursing is learning the psychology of the Doctor that is scheduled on any given shift and to talk about how these things aren't one-off situations. They literally come to the surface every. single. shift. The idea was to reveal how healthcare isn't a luxury, but it's a *necessity* where year-after-year, the job becomes more of a service industry combined with endless charting—even on a small event just to make sure you don't get fired. The frustration is mounting.

I wish I had the answer to things, but I don't. In the military, I would tell my soldiers not to come to me with problems but to come to me with solutions. And here I am, maybe the hypocrite for violating my own advice. In the years I witnessed and experienced all the mounting frustrations, I did indeed put a great amount of thought into what could be done differently and typically came up blank. The answer always remained foggy but did seem to swirl around how things would need to change on a mass scale. So the "answer" turned into "reach out to the masses" in my own way. Not like the majority of what is currently out on the market.

If nothing else, I encourage you to sit down with any Nurse you know and ask for *their* stories. Hell, more than half the time I bring up the topic of my endeavor (this book) to another Nurse, they launch into a tirade of their own experience, some of it is a shared nursing collective but more often than not other Nurses will bring up things that made me think *they* are the ones that should've written a book like this, not me. So, talk to a Nurse you know. You will have a night full of mixed emotions from the shock value of hearing about massive traumatic incidents of patients that come to the ER with nearly every bone in their body broken, internal bleeding, and the roulette of efforts from multiple people that all somehow end up on the same page to help the person live to see another day. Or the mixed emotions of working a code for 45 minutes on someone's grandmother after the family made the decision to overturn her DNR in the heat of the moment because "she's a fighter."

You'll get the common themes of a small group of red faced, neck vein bulging, furious people yelling at the triage Nurse because they have been waiting for hours to be taken into an ER Room. But you will also get endearing stories, like a little girl that took comfort in having a Nurse that also had freckles, proudly proclaiming that they are Angel Kisses.

You'll hear details and tales of patients' last moments like blood that rolled across the entirety of the ER Bay when the last ditch effort of the ER Trauma team was to crack a patient's chest wide open, revealing a knife completely severing his heart from his aorta. Followed up with arguable poetic justice of how the knife ended up there because roughly an hour ago the patient was beating on his spouse who then, through the fury of fists coming at her, grabbed the first thing that her hand gripped and slammed it into the patient's chest.

You'll hear takes of "I can't believe that's medicine" like when the Urologist gets consulted to the ER for a difficult urinary catheter placement, and they unroll their tools of the trade like their Dexter Morgan's kill kit. Followed up with a Dark Ages description of the process required to insert a urinary catheter and drain the patient's bladder.

You'll get wild tales of Nurses tackling naked patients in the middle of a mental health crisis that got spooked by their hallucinations and ran through the ER. Tales of skin flakes dusting the air when a patient's socks are removed to assess a potential broken foot.

Many Nurses also have stories of getting assaulted by patients for every reason from an acutely emotional father who was lashing out over the hospital team ending resuscitation efforts on his adolescent son all the way to full grown adults who immediately move to violence after they get Narcan to reverse a drug overdose.

But that's all just the 99% of the gig . . . remember the 1%? *That's* really why I wanted to write this book. *That's* why, for all the shitty shifts and night-after-night chaos of it all, I know there is still a reason for walking through those doors each night—a reason that is far bigger than myself and *much* bigger than any sort of "calling" I felt for my life. The 1% that reminds any Nurse of why they signed up for this fucking circus is enough to keep them there *juuust* long enough. And "just long enough" might be 50 years (God bless those Nurses) or "just long enough" might be 5 months. All I know is that if we keep going at this rate, more Nurses will trend toward the latter. And I sincerely hope that's not the case, because if a Nurse tosses in the towel after his or her 15th month of time served, they'll never know who they could have helped or saved during their 16th.

Maybe . . . *maybe* this book helps those Nurses *regain* a pulse on why they signed up for this, and what it takes to hang on a little longer. And maybe . . . *maybe* this book helps patients *get* a pulse, for the first time in your life, on what really happens behind those hallowed doors—the good, the bad, and God-forsaken ugly.

And if you are one of those patients, just sit down with a Nurse sometime, have a beer—no more, no less—and get ready to hear some stories that you'll have a hard time believing. Then again, if you've made it to this point in the book, I guess you should have a better pulse of what's really going on out here.

Cheers.

ACKNOWLEDGMENTS

While the introduction is irritatingly true about the "look at how cool I am" nursing texts that currently make up the market, I actually began this book as a project to deal with frustrations of the job myself. After any particularly emotional shift in any direction: angering, inspiring, sorrowful, etc. with no book or show to accurately relate to, I would immediately open up a writing document and brain dump everything onto the digital pages. They read like the ramblings of a madman. But they accumulated.

My thanks is heavily to ZR, MR, KW, & BB who not only read the sheer ugliness of those writings but somehow saw through abundant swearing that I vomited all over the digital pages but also gave truly constructive criticism and supported my efforts forward.

Additionally, my thanks to Will. The man with the heart of gold who very likely did not understand the full weight of what he was getting into when he agreed to help turn my jargon and rambling into more than a message but a book worth reading. His skill in translating people's stories to reach further than their immediate circle is impressive.

Lastly, a special sort of thanks to all those dumbass "HEROES WORK HERE" banners that kept the embers of my anger from going dark every time I began and ended each shift.

ABOUT THE AUTHOR

Before his time as a nurse, Adam Rozendaal spent 10 years in the Army as a Medic. He was twice overseas—two 12-month deployments to Kosovo from 2007-2008, and Kuwait/Iraq from 2011-2012. Seeing a natural bridge between life as a medic and nurse, Adam transitioned to life as a full time Critical Care Nurse in 2012 where he worked in the Emergency Room until 2020. At that time, he transitioned into the ICU. Adam now serves as a travel nurse who takes contracts in either department.

Adam has worked mostly in Colorado, but also in Oregon, Oklahoma, Maryland, and now Tennessee.

in 2019 Adam was diagnoses with a form of Non-Hodgkin Lymphoma (Anaplastic Large Cell Lymphoma). He had pain and symptoms for almost six months before getting a diagnosis, then five months of chemo. After a three week hospital stay, he was released after his first chemo treatment. He celebrated his 3-Year Remission Anniversary in July of 2022.

In his free time, he's hiking trails or letting the minutes pass like hours at a cafe with a cup of coffee.